THE ROLE OF ANDROGENS IN MEN'S HEALTH

A Guide for Healthcare Professionals

Dr Geoff Hackett
MD FRCPI MRCGP

Distributed with permission as a service to medicine
by Bayer Schering Pharma

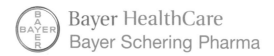

Bayer HealthCare
Bayer Schering Pharma

THE ROLE OF ANDROGENS IN MEN'S HEALTH

A Guide for Healthcare Professionals

Published in the UK by:

National Services for Health Improvement

Nucleus@The Bridge

London Science and Business Park

Brunel Way, Dartford DA1 5GA

Copyright 2009 National Services for Health Improvement

Printed in the UK by Stephens and George Ltd

ISBN 978-0-9560921-1-3

About the author

Dr Geoff Hackett MD FRCPI MRCGP has been a family physician for over 29 years and a consultant in Sexual Medicine/ Urology since 1994. He obtained his MD at Keele University on the management of male sexual problems in primary care in 2000 and also won the Charles Oliver Hawthorn Award for research in 1986, from the BMA, and the Duke of Edinburgh Prize in Sports Medicine in 1993.

From 2005-2007, he was the President of the British Society for Sexual Medicine and has been on the Scientific Committee of the ESSM since 2002. Geoff has published over 40 papers and chapters on Sexual Medicine.

Introduction

For over 30 years, physicians have been aware of the importance of hormonal changes with ageing (*Figure 1.1*). Testosterone levels fall progressively in men from the age of 30 (*Table 1.2*) but few primary care physicians ever consider measurement of testosterone in men presenting with symptoms, such as tiredness, sweating, poor concentration, altered mood or depression. Androgen therapy has been viewed with suspicion, often perceived as a form of non evidence based quackery practiced by private Harley Street physicians. Others have felt that it is inappropriate to interfere with normal ageing processes or that we must heed warnings from our enthusiasm for HRT in females, most likely in terms of long-term detrimental effects on the prostate. However, multiple large scale studies have shown the beneficial effects of androgen therapy in hypogonadal men combined with evidence of long-term safety.

Unfortunately, abuse of testosterone and anabolic steroids in sport has led to many misconceptions about therapy. Essentially, all endocrine deficiencies require replacement within physiological levels and large or inappropriate use is associated with risks. This means that the summary of product characteristics (SPC) of testosterone medications has to mention symptoms related to possible abuse and this frequently causes unnecessary alarm.

As much of primary care management involves the prevention of cardiovascular events, the life expectancy of men has improved considerably over the last 30 years (*Figure 1.2*). Patients would ideally like to enjoy a higher quality of life in these additional years, essentially extending the years of middle life rather than senility. Issues such as the prevention of osteoporosis or dementia in ageing men become more important as longevity is enhanced. These are issues that we rarely discuss with ageing men.

The development of guidelines[1] in the management of erectile dysfunction has meant that all newly presenting patients be checked for morning levels of total testosterone. The correction of low levels can restore erectile function, both alone and in conjunction with other therapies, and also enhance levels of sexual desire in ageing men. This has been the main driving force behind a new level of interest in hypogonadism in ageing men.

In the following chapters, the author explores recent research in andrology; Chapter 1 addresses the accurate diagnosis of androgen deficiency, and the current evidence based management of endocrine problems in the ageing male. Chapter 2 explores in depth recent research into the important associations between testosterone deficiency, type 2 diabetes and metabolic syndrome. Chapter 3 reviews the diagnostic criteria and Chapter 4 evaluates current therapies. Chapter 5 assesses the importance of desire disorders in men and in particular the role of androgens and prescribed drugs.

Chapter 6 consists of a series of case studies from the author's clinical practice together with key learning points, as, in his experience, this is often the best way of teaching sexual medicine.

Contents

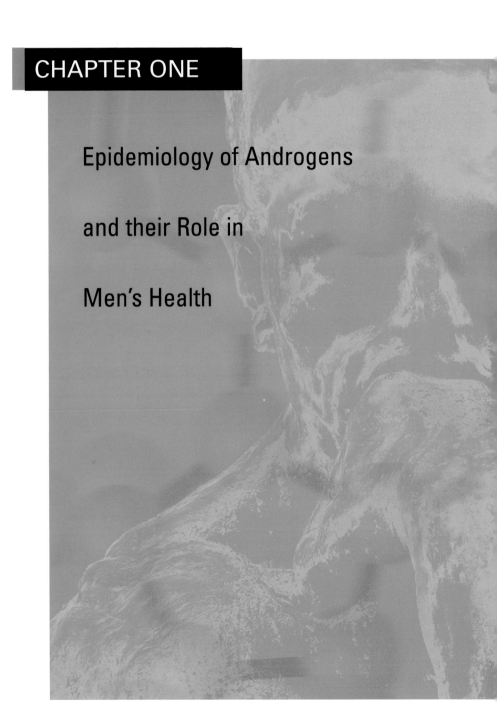

CHAPTER ONE

Epidemiology of Androgens

and their Role in

Men's Health

Figure 1.1 Longitudinal changes in serum testosterone levels

(Morley JE et al[2,] 1997)

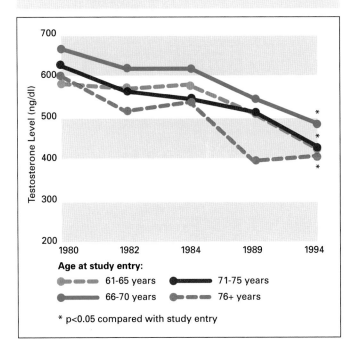

Age at study entry:

● ─ ─ ─ 61-65 years   ●▬▬▬▬ 71-75 years

●───── 66-70 years   ●─ ─ ─ 76+ years

* p<0.05 compared with study entry

Table 1.1 Age and hormones[2]

Age and hormones	
• Testosterone decreases	• Thyroxin declines
• Growth Hormone (GH) decreases 14% per decade	• Antidiuretic Hormone (ADH) declines
• Interstitial Growth factor (IGF-1) declines (related to GH)	• No age related Estradiol change
• DHEA-S decreases 22% per decade	• Melatonin decreases with age
• Slight increase in Sex Hormone Binding Globulin (SHBG)	• Leptin (produced by adipocytes) increase with age

Figure 1.2 Life expectancy for men and women *(A White, 2004³)*

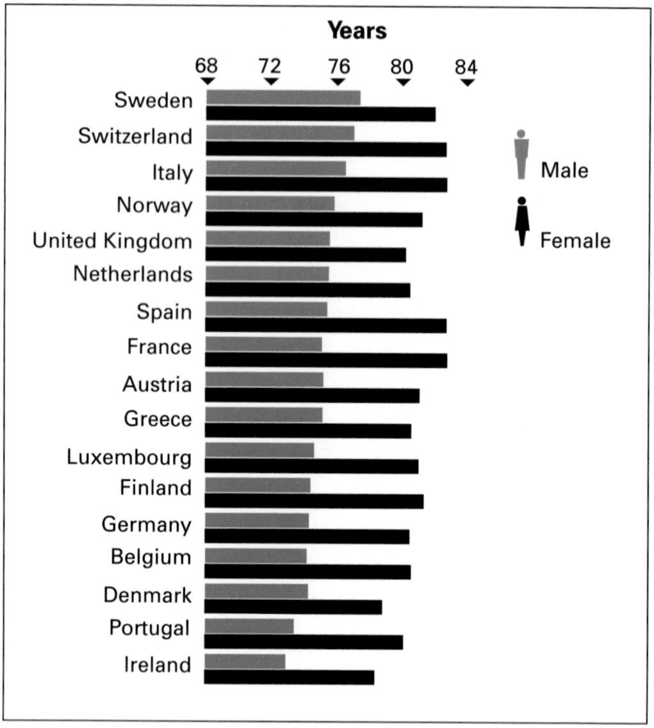

Years

| | 68 | 72 | 76 | 80 | 84 |

Sweden
Switzerland
Italy   Male
Norway
United Kingdom   Female
Netherlands
Spain
France
Austria
Greece
Luxembourg
Finland
Germany
Belgium
Denmark
Portugal
Ireland

Definitions

Several terms have been used for the condition of androgen deficiency in ageing males, but Late Onset Hypogonadism (LOH) or Testosterone Deficiency Syndrome (TDS) is currently preferred. Andropause is a clinical condition characterised by partial androgen deficiency in systemic blood flow. However, men with apparently low normal testosterone can have andropausic symptoms. These symptoms can be attributed to a decreased genomic sensitivity to testosterone or its active metabolites in the target organs of androgens. The term andropause is not currently fashionable, as it suggests that there is a male equivalent to the female menopause. Other terms include Androgen deficiency of the ageing male (ADAM) or Partial Androgen Deficiency of the Ageing Male (PADAM) or Partial Androgen Deficiency.

The current BSSM (British Society for Sexual Medicine), ISSAM (International Society for Study of the Aging Male), EAU (European Urology Association)[1,73,44] definition is:

A biochemical syndrome associated with advancing age and characterised by a deficiency in serum androgen levels with or without a decreased genomic sensitivity to androgens. It may result in significant alterations in the quality of life and adversely affect the function of multiple organ systems.

This state of hypogonadism causes a global decrease in energy and a decrease in the feeling of well-being. It also causes a change in sexual function and has other endocrine and metabolic repercussions. These can affect bones, muscles, and lipids, as well as cognitive function.

The appearance of symptoms must be confirmed with testing to determine whether the patient is indeed experiencing a decrease in testosterone production. The differential diagnosis will depend on the physician's identification and assessment of clinical symptoms, as well as testing for low testosterone.

Testosterone is present in three main fractions:

- Free (2-3%)

- Albumin bound (20-40%)

- And tightly bound to Sex Hormone Binding Globulin (SHBG) (60-80%)

Non SHBG bound testosterone is considered to be the biologically active fragment, referred to as Bioavailable Testosterone (BAT).

Hypogonadism and testosterone replacement therapy

Androgen deficiency in the adult male becomes more common with increasing age[2] but its management remains controversial. As well as sexual dysfunction, androgen deficiency is associated with osteoporosis, dyslipidaemia, metabolic syndrome and depression. Far from being a benign consequence of ageing, it has important and unwanted metabolic consequences, and is a significant cause of increased cardiovascular risk. Several large scale studies, notably the Massachusetts Male Ageing Study (MMAS)[4] and the HIM study[5], have suggested links with obesity, metabolic syndrome and approximately double the risk of developing type 2 diabetes. As yet, there are no long-term studies to suggest that correcting androgen deficiency will mitigate this risk but ongoing research will, hopefully, answer these questions.

MMAS studied 3,518 men for over 17 years, dividing men into groups by increments of 7 nmol/litre (200 ng/dl) of total testosterone. The investigators found that men with low total testosterone (T) levels are nearly twice as likely to die from all causes and cardiovascular disease compared to men with a normal T level. However, when it came to cancer-related deaths, a low T level conveyed a three-fold higher risk of death from all cancer.

The age adjusted Hazard Ratios for men with total T<200 ng/dL (7 nmol/L) vs. men with total T of 410-509 ng/dL (14 nmol/L)[6] were:

- 1.93 or two-fold for all mortalities (p=0.03)

- 3.30 or three-fold for cancer death (p=0.03)

- 1.93 or two-fold for CVD death (p= 0.028)

The findings from this large scale study with long-term follow-up of 17 years have received little discussion, in comparison with many shorter term follow-up studies in hypertension. A three-fold increase in all cancer risks in hypogonadal men suggests considerable reassurance regarding any risk of prostate cancer.

Shores[7] in 2004, Loughlin[8] in 2008 and the Rotterdam study[18] showed strong associations between low total testosterone and mortality, equating to a 68% additional risk between the men with a total testosterone of less than 8 nmol/L and those in the normal range *(Table 1.2)*. It is of interest that, in a similar age group of over 9,000 men followed up for over five years,

Thompson et al[19] found the risk of coronary heart disease (CHD) associated with current cigarette smoking to be 46%, similar to the risk associated with incident erectile dysfunction (ED). Although drawing conclusions between different studies is fraught with difficulties, it could be postulated that having a serum total testosterone less than 8 nmol/L[20] carries a greater risk of early death than smoking. Ma et al showed that the presence of ED in type 2 diabetic males was a stronger predictor of CHD events than HbA1c, lipids or microalbuminuria. Gazzaruso[21] showed that the severity of ED predicted the

Table 1.2 Increased all cause mortality associated with hypogonadism

(Shores M et al.)

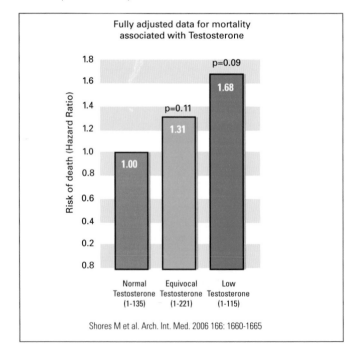

Shores M et al. Arch. Int. Med. 2006 166: 1660-1665

severity of atheroma found at coronary angiography in type 2 diabetes. Strong associations with low Testosterone and ED, particularly in T2D, constitute a compelling case for inclusion as markers in the routine risk management of CHD.

Whilst there is much current debate as to whether treatment should be based on total, free, or bioavailable testosterone, it should be remembered that all these longitudinal studies quantified risk on the basis of total testosterone.

Testosterone and cardiovascular disease

Pre-menopausal women suffer significantly less from cardiovascular disease than men and traditionally this has been explained by the presumed beneficial effects of oestrogen on lipid profiles and the relatively detrimental effects of testosterone[9]. Patients with CHD tend to have lower testosterone levels[10] *(Figures 1.3 & 1.4)* than normal and levels of testosterone fall after acute myocardial infarction.

Cross-sectional studies in men show a positive correlation between FT (Free testosterone) levels and HDL (high density lipoprotein) cholesterol and a negative correlation with fibrinogen, plasminogen activator inhibitor-1 (PAI-1) and insulin levels, as well as coronary artery disease, but not cardiovascular mortality.[10]

TRT (testosterone replacement therapy) produces a modest reduction in BP of the order of 4–5mmHg[13], and:

- Minimally lowers total cholesterol[12] (seen more often in younger patients, not those with LOH)

- Minimally lowers HDL cholesterol[12]

- In 14 out of 15 published studies, produced a mean 15% reduction in LDL (low density lipoprotein)[13]

- Shows slight reductions of apolipoproteins A and B7[14]

Figure 1.3 Testosterone levels and CHD *(English[10])*

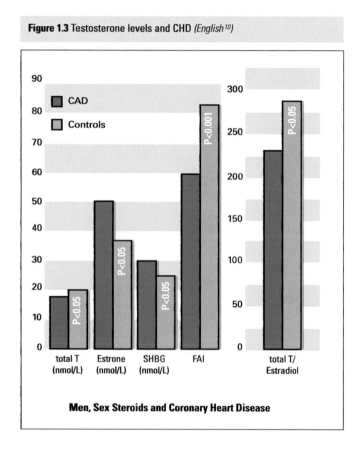

Men, Sex Steroids and Coronary Heart Disease

The MRFIT[15] study showed that hypogonadal men had slightly increased triglycerides and HDL.

Trials have shown pharmacological doses of testosterone to relax coronary arteries when injected intraluminally[16,17] and to produce modest but consistent improvement in exercise-induced angina and reverse associated ECG changes[16,17].

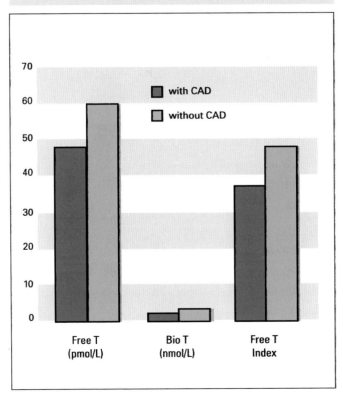

Figure 1.4 Androgens in men with or without angiographic CAD
(English, 2000[10])

TRT has also been shown to reduce fibrinogen to levels similar to fibrates[14].

The consensus is that the overall effect of testosterone on these metabolic changes is a net benefit in terms of cardiovascular risk![2]

The most compelling data linking low testosterone levels with increased mortality were provided by the EPIC study in Norfolk[22]. This was a nested case-control study comparing 825 men without CVD and cancer at baseline and who died in the follow-up period of up to 10 years, with 1,489 men who were still alive. Baseline testosterone levels were inversely related to deaths due to all causes, CVD and malignancy after controlling for the usual confounders. Mean hip–waist ratio, prevalence of cigarette smoking and DM (diabetes mellitus) were all significantly higher in men who died from cardiovascular causes (p values of <0.01, <0.001 and <0.001 respectively). These men also had significantly higher mean systolic BP (p<0.001), plasma triglycerides (p<0.001), BMI (p<0.01), total cholesterol (p=0.01) and LDL:HDL cholesterol ratio (p<0.01) at baseline.

Men were categorised by quartile of serum testosterone levels. These were <12.5 (n=569), 12.5-15.6 (n=595), 15.7-19.6 (n=568), >19.6 nmol/L (n=582). Testosterone levels were significantly inversely related to BMI, (p<0.001), waist-hip ratio (p<0.001), triglycerides (p<0.001) and prevalence of DM (p<0.001) and positively related to total cholesterol (p<0.001),

LDL-cholesterol (p<0.001), HDL-cholesterol (p<0.001) and cigarette smoking (p<0.01).

Cardiovascular mortality was shown to be independently related to testosterone levels with OR (odds ratio) (95% CIs given) for each quartile being 1, 0.89, 0.6 and 0.53 respectively, with a p value for the trend of <0.01after adjustments for the recognised CVD risk factors. Cardiovascular mortality was assessed before and after the exclusion of those who had died in the first two years. Before exclusion the ORs were 0.83 (p<0.01) and 0.76 (p<0.010) after adjustments for age and covariates respectively. The corresponding ratios after the exclusion of those who died in the first two years were 0.85 (p=0.02) and 0.79 (p=0.02) respectively.

An increase of 6 nmol/L of testosterone was associated with a multivariate adjusted OR of 0.81 (p<0.01) for overall mortality. Thus, the death rate was decreased by 14% irrespective of whether the patient was above or below 65 years. The authors noted that the relationships of baseline testosterone levels to cardiovascular mortality was unchanged after adjustment for the classic risk factors, so that the protective effect of testosterone may be through modulating inflammatory markers or haemostatic factors, or via improved endothelial function and coronary vasodilation[75].

The findings of the EPIC study were reproduced in the Rancho Bernardo study[23]. The study comprised 794 men aged between 50-91 years. The median TT and bioavailable testosterone were 10.2 nmol/L and 2.5 nmol/L respectively. The average duration of follow-up was 11.8 years. Men whose TT was in the lowest quartile (<8 nmol/L) were 40% (HR 1.4, p=0.002 after adjusting for age, BMI, waist-hip ratio, alcohol use, current smoking and exercise) more likely to die from all causes than those with higher levels. Low TT also predicted an increased risk of CV mortality (HR 1.38) as did low bioavailable testosterone levels (HR 1.36). The effect was still present after excluding deaths which occurred in the first five years for both TT and bioavailable testosterone levels. For total testosterone, the HR was 1.73 and for bioavailable testosterone, 1.39 (p values not stated). In this study, lower TT levels were associated with central obesity and established CVD risk factors (insulin and insulin resistance glycaemia, lipid profile, blood pressure) and emerging risk factors (leptin, adiponectin and CRP - C reactive protein) [*Laughlin et al 2008*][8].

These two important studies from well respected Investigators show that cardiovascular mortality and low testosterone levels are clearly associated, and that low testosterone levels can be regarded as an independent, predictive risk factor for CV mortality.

Other studies supporting the association between TDS and CVD are:

1. Low TT (r = -0.36, p = 0.008) and free testosterone levels (r = -0.49, p<0.001) were inversely correlated to CAD even after adjusting for age and adiposity.[24]

2. Men with angiographically proven CAD (coronary artery disease) had significantly lower testosterone levels compared to controls (p<0.01) and there was a significant inverse relationship between the degree of CAD and TT (total testosterone) levels (r = -0.52, p<0.01).[25]

3. Nearly 25% of men presenting for coronary angiography had testosterone levels in the low hypogonadal range and some 50% had a TT of less than 11 nmol/L.[26]

Osteoporosis, fracture and risk of falls

The prevalence of osteoporosis in men over 50 is 4-6%, and hypogonadism, particularly with onset in younger men, is an acknowledged risk factor (in around 20% of all male cases) with white men at greater risk (7%) than black (5%), or Hispanic American men (3%)[27]. The importance of LOH in terms of osteoporosis is less clear but 30% of all hip fractures over 75 occur in men (*Figures 1.5 and 1.6*).

This becomes more important when population data show that by age 75 there are around 60 living men for every 100 living women[3]. The morbidity and mortality of osteoporotic fractures are significantly higher in men than women[27] *(Table 1.3)*.

In terms of both primary and secondary prevention of osteoporosis, men are largely ignored, with the perception being that osteoporotic fracture is almost exclusively a problem in post-menopausal women *(Figures 1.5 and 1.6, Table 1.3)*.

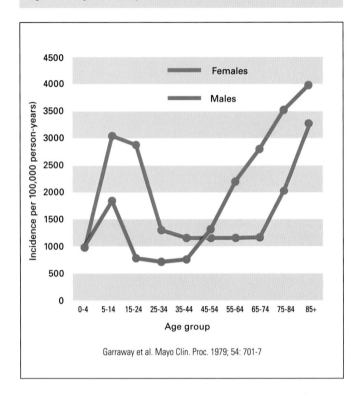

Figure 1.5 Age and sex-specific incidence of all limb fractures

Garraway et al. Mayo Clin. Proc. 1979; 54: 701-7

Current NICE (National Institute of Health and Clinical Excellence) guidance[28] on osteoporosis concentrates exclusively on women and there is currently no guidance for men, although hypogonadism is frequently quoted as a major risk factor. NICE guidance on prostate cancer[29] does stress the importance of osteoporosis treatment in men on androgen ablation therapy.

Figure 1.6 Osteoporotic fracture incidence

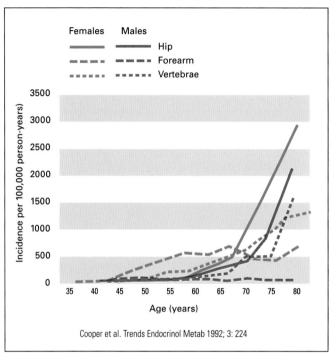

Cooper et al. Trends Endocrinol Metab 1992; 3: 224

Table 1.3 Mortality after major types of osteoporotic fracture in men and women

(Cooper et al. Trends Endocrinol Metab 1992; 3: 224)

5 year prospective cohort study		
Age standardised mortality ratio		
Fracture	Women	Men
Proximal femur	2.2	3.2
Vertebral	1.7	2.4
Other major	1.9	2.2
Other minor	0.8	1.5

The importance of androgen deficiency in relation to osteoporosis is more significant as hypogonadism has been associated with cognitive impairment[33] and risk of falls in the elderly[43,44], increasing fracture risk. The MINOS[43] study looked at 1,040 French men aged 51–85 and the MrOS[44] study in the US studied 2,587 community based men aged 65 to 99 and concluded that men with a bioavailable testosterone in the lower quartile had a 40% additional risk of fall. The effect was most apparent in the 65 to 69 age group, and in men aged over 80 testosterone levels were not associated with falls. The authors concluded that *"these results provide additional justification for trials of testosterone in older men and should aid in the design of those studies"*. Despite these findings, Kiebzak[45] et al in a review of 363 patients admitted for osteoporotic fracture (110 men and 253 women) only 4.5% of men v 27% of women had prior treatment. The 12 month mortality for men was 32% compared with 17% for women. At 12 month follow-up of survivors, 27% of men versus 71% of women were taking treatment (usually only calcium and vitamin D). Eleven per cent of men versus 27% of women received follow-up bone density assessment.

A recent long-term study on the effects of testosterone treatment showed that Bone Mineral Density (BMD) continues to increase in the lumbar spine after 18 to 30 months of treatment *(Figure 1.7)*[32]. Meta-regression analysis performed at the lumbar spine and femoral neck revealed a significant effect of TRT, and pooled results from eight Randomised Clinical Trials (RCTs)[31] found that testosterone had a moderate effect on bone resorption markers. Until now no adequately powered trial has yet explored the impact of therapy on hip and vertebral fracture.

Figure 1.7 Effects of long-term TRT on bone density
(Wang et al, 2004[32])

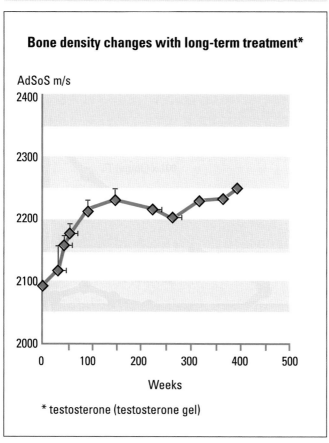

Bone density changes with long-term treatment*

AdSoS m/s

Weeks

* testosterone (testosterone gel)

Cognitive function

There is evidence that hypogonadism is associated with decreased cognitive function and that testosterone administration enhances performance on spatial cognition and mathematical reasoning[33]. In the MMAS[4], there was no evidence that older age was associated with testosterone in terms of spatial ability, working memory and speed/attention when adjusted for age and co-variants. However, in the 10-year longitudinal assessment of multiple cognitive domains, higher free testosterone predicted better scores on visual and verbal memory, visual-spatial functioning, visual motor scanning and a reduced rate of longitudinal decline in visual memory[34]. Studies consistently show that T therapy improves mood, energy and well-being in younger men, but the effects tend to be less clear in ageing men[35]. Nevertheless, benefits are consistently clear in a subset of ageing men with manifest low testosterone[36] (*see Figure 1.8*).

Mood and depression

Symptoms associated with low testosterone are diminished energy, reduced vitality or well-being, increased fatigue, depressed mood, impaired cognition, decreased muscle mass and strength, diminished bone density and anaemia. The lifetime prevalence of depression, at 24%, is known to be three times higher in type 2 diabetics than the general population and the most commonly cited reason is the burden of co-morbidities in

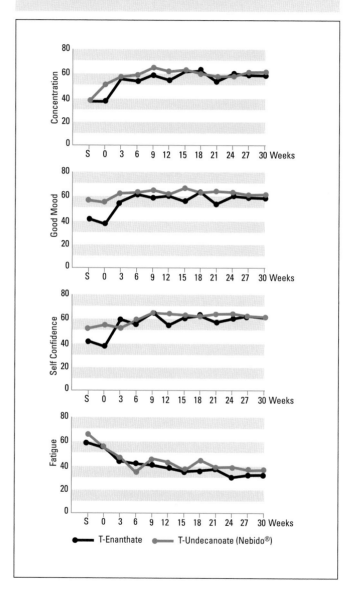

Epidemiology of Androgens and their Role in Men's Health

diabetes[37]. None of the papers reviewed in meta analysis of 42 studies in 2001[38] considered androgen status, despite the obvious overlap in symptoms between hypogonadism and depression. Depression was found to be more common in male than in female type 2 diabetics, the reverse of the non-diabetic population, suggesting a possible role for testosterone. The 2008 UK GP contract[39] has set a target for 90% of type 2 diabetics to be screened for depression with guidance as to how the burden of detected depression should be managed with increase in prescribing of SSRI antidepressants and CBT, (cognitive behavioural therapy) acknowledging that these measures have not been shown to improve glycaemic control[50]. Kapoor and others[40,41,42,43] have demonstrated that the symptoms of hypogonadism, insulin resistance and HbA1c improved when the testosterone deficiency was corrected.

Testosterone therapy is clearly associated with general mood elevating effects and some studies have shown associations between low testosterone and depression. Although low testosterone has been shown to predict incident depression in ageing men and a significant relationship between androgen receptor polymorphism, only two of nine RCTs (randomised clinical trials)[44] have shown a significant improvement on depression scores in ageing men compared with placebo. Combined therapy with anti-depressants has been shown to be superior to anti-depressant plus placebo in a group of younger men with refractory depression[44].

Figure 1.9 Relationship between hypogonadism and incident depression[34]

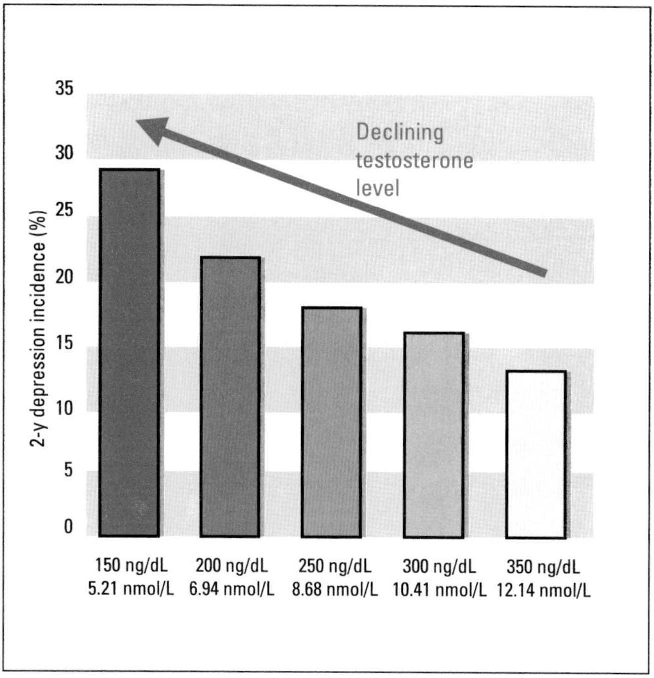
35
30
25
20
15
10
5
0
2-y depression incidence (%)
Declining
testosterone
level
150 ng/dL
5.21 nmol/L
200 ng/dL
6.94 nmol/L
250 ng/dL
8.68 nmol/L
300 ng/dL
10.41 nmol/L
350 ng/dL
12.14 nmol/L

Testosterone and Alzheimer's disease

Men are relatively protected from Alzheimer's disease compared with women. There is evidence that androgens confer protection from Alzheimer's disease in their own right and a recent study found a link between cognitive functioning and bioavailable testosterone[45]. Testosterone therapy has been shown to improve mood and quality of life in men with Alzheimer's disease despite cognitive improvement failing to reach clinical significance[46]. The conclusion from these studies would be that free testosterone should be monitored in cases of Alzheimer's disease and a therapeutic trial may be appropriate in many cases[46].

Polycythaemia

Testosterone is a physiological stimulus of erythrocytosis[48]. The mild anaemia related to old age has been postulated as being due to testosterone deficiency. Testosterone therapy usually corrects this anaemia[49] but smokers or patients with COPD (chronic obstructive pulmonary disease) or heart failure are at greater risk of polycythaemia. Risks are greater with the older intramuscular preparations compared with newer transdermal delivery or the newer long-acting intramuscular injection. There has been no evidence of increased thrombotic episodes in any of the published studies[48]. Guidelines suggest that the blood count should be checked within three months of therapy and annually thereafter[1].

Endocrine aspects of Sexual Function

Endocrine disorders may have a significant effect on sexual function[1]. The resolution of endocrine abnormalities might also lead to the resolution of co-existing sexual dysfunction. As current guidelines recommend that a measurement of morning testosterone, fasting lipids and blood glucose are mandatory in new cases of ED, hypogonadism will be detected as part of routine management[1]. A second measurement should be taken before 11am, along with SHBG (for calculated free testosterone), prolactin, LH and FSH. Hyperprolactinaemia (levels up to 900 nmol/L) can be related to stress but levels above this need further investigation and endocrinology referral to exclude a pituitary adenoma[1].

Thyroid function should be checked if symptoms of hyper or hypothyroidism are present. Hypothyroidism is associated with retarded ejaculation and hyperthyroidism is a treatable cause of premature ejaculation (if detected)[47]. The advice of an endocrinologist is necessary where there is doubt as to the cause and appropriate management of the disorder. Although current guidelines do not suggest measurement of thyroid function in all cases of ED, testing is inexpensive and correcting the underlying abnormality may prove curative[1].

Androgens act at several sites in the sexual response system: within the CNS, peripheral nitrergic nerves, and corpora cavernosa. Androgens play an important role in up-regulation of the nitric oxide-cyclic GMP pathway, preserving the oxygenation of cavernosal smooth muscle[51]. Loss of androgen is associated, experimentally, with deterioration in morphology and function of cavernosal smooth muscle[51]. Several studies have shown improvement in erectile function with androgen replacement alone, particularly when other risk factors, such as diabetes and hypertension are absent. The SPC (summary of product characteristics) of the topical treatments state that *"testosterone is not a treatment for impotence"* but this is to discourage the practice of prescribing testosterone for all patients without appropriate investigation[1].

Androgen deficiency may affect sexual interest, erections, and responsiveness to PDE5 (phosphodiesterase type 5) inhibitors[51]. In most of the clinical trials of oral therapies for ED, patients with untreated hypogonadism were excluded and therefore quoted responses from such clinical trials should not be expected when men are treated without assessment of androgen status[51].

Low testosterone is the most common reason for sub-optimal response to PDE5. Kalinchenko[51] showed that in a group of sildenafil non-responders, the mean total testosterone was 6.9 nmol/L versus 18.6 in a group of responders *(Table 1.5)*. Shabsigh[53] et al demonstrated that patients previously non-responsive to sildenafil could be salvaged when low testosterone levels (less than 14 nmol/L) were restored to normal with the use of transdermal testosterone *(Table 1.6)*. These findings, which have been reproduced in many subsequent studies, were potentially the most relevant clinical indication for testosterone prescribing, as patients failing to respond to a PDE5 inhibitor would be reluctant to move to injection therapy if another option exists.

Table 1.5 Different testosterone levels in diabetic responders and non-responders to sildenafil (Viagra®)

	Viagra non-responders n=120	Viagra responders n=100	
	Mean ± SD	Mean ± SD	p value
Total testosterone	6.9 ± 1.3	18.6 ± 1.2	<0.001
(nmol/L)	(4.5–9.6)	(14.3–29.1)	

Table 1.6 12 wk testosterone therapy converts sildenafil 100mg non-responders to responders in men with hypogonadism (tt<14 nmol/L) and erectile dysfunction

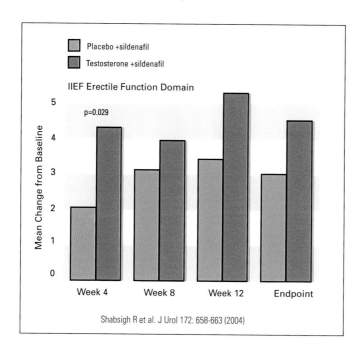

Shabsigh R et al. J Urol 172: 658-663 (2004)

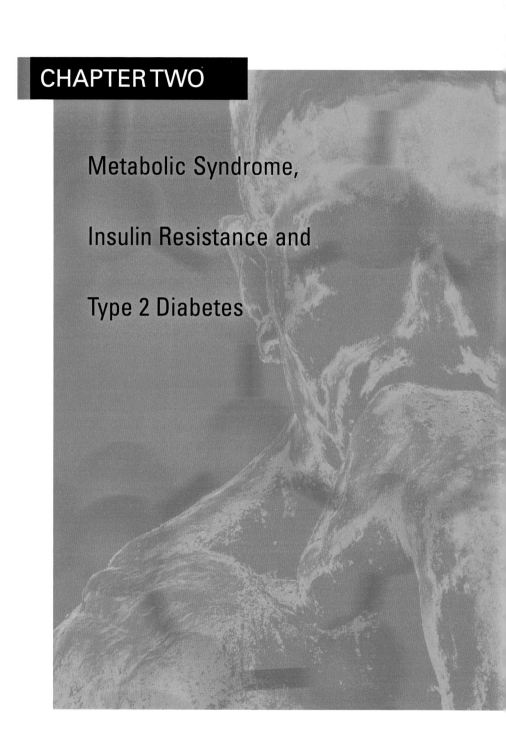

CHAPTER TWO

Metabolic Syndrome,

Insulin Resistance and

Type 2 Diabetes

Studies have shown an inverse relationship between serum testosterone and fasting blood glucose and insulin levels[54]. Both hyperinsulinaemia and low testosterone have been shown to predict the development of type 2 diabetes (T2D), and testosterone therapy has been shown to reduce insulin resistance in obese and elderly men[8]. Hypogonadism is associated with increased visceral obesity, and TRT has been shown in elderly and obese males to reduce visceral obesity and increase lean muscle mass.

Hypogonadism appears to be a common feature of the metabolic syndrome (*Table 2.1*)[5]. Whether the hypogonadism develops as a consequence of the metabolic syndrome or whether the hypogonadism is involved in the pathogenesis is unclear, but current evidence, particularly from the MMAS[12,] suggests that low testosterone and low SHBG,[55] predict the development of metabolic syndrome and type 2 diabetes.

Women with T2D or metabolic syndrome characteristically have low SHBG and high free testosterone[56]. Insulin therapy frequently results in weight gain and metformin has been shown to produce modest reduction of total testosterone[51].

Table 2.1 Hypogonadism and metabolic syndrome – the HIM study[5]

Hypogonadism and metabolic syndrome – the HIM study

- 2,165 men >45 in 95 US practices attending for routine appointments with primary care physicians (87% acceptance rate)
- Study conducted Nov 03 – Feb 04
- Bloods taken between 8am and noon for Total Testosterone (TT) (by Radio-Immunoassay), Free Testosterone (FT) (equilibrium dialysis), Bioavailable Testosterone (BAT) and SHBG
- Co-morbid conditions, weight, BMI, BP
- Hypogonadism <10.4 nmol/l   38.7% by TT

                             40.0% by FT

                             45.0% by BAT

Table 1.3 Ratios of hypogonadism with co-morbid conditions [5]

HIM study (2,165 men)	Prevalence	Range	Odds ratio
Obesity	52.4	(47.9 – 56.9)	2.38
Diabetes	50	(45.5 – 54.5)	2.09
Hypertension	42.4	(39.6 – 45.2)	1.84
Hyperlipidaemia	40.4	(37.6 – 43.3)	1.47
Osteoporosis	44.4	(25.5 – 64.7)	1.41
BPH	41.3	(36.4 – 46.2)	1.29

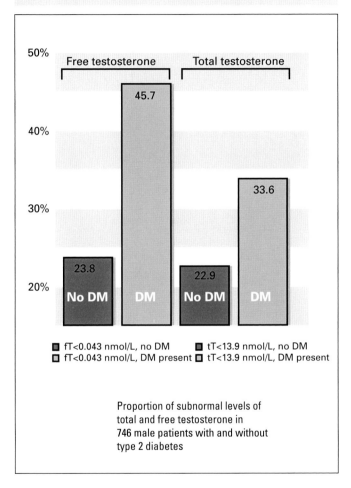

The precise interaction between insulin resistance and hypogonadism is, as yet, unclear but Caprio[58] summarised the links between obesity and low testosterone (*Figures 2.2 and 2.3*).

Figure 2.2 Adipose tissue and testosterone

(Caprio et al, 2001)

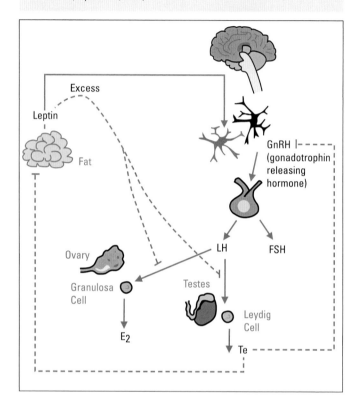

In obese males: levels of testosterone are reduced in proportion to degree of obesity[58]

♦ Leptin is produced by adipose tissue[58]

♦ Leptin inhibits secretion of testosterone and is a causal factor of LOH in obese males

♦ Leptin is the best predictive factor of testosterone deficit in ageing males[58]

Figure 2.3 Testosterone and obesity – the hypogonadal-obesity cycle
(Cohen PG, 1999)

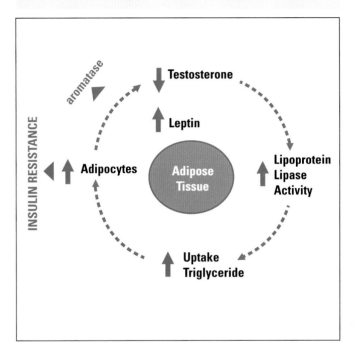

♦ Testosterone treatment in ageing males reduces obesity[58]

The author has completed an audit of 488 type 2 diabetics in primary care practices in Burtwood, Lichfield and Tamworth, the BLT study[60]. The important findings were a significant difference in BMI, waist circumference, HbA1c and SHIM (Sexual Health Inventory for Men), a well validated assessment tool for erectile dysfunction. Results are summarised in *Tables 2.3, 2.4 and 2.5, 2.6, 2.7.*

The 2004 GP contract and subsequent revisions for 2008/9[61] put strong emphasis on T2D as a target priority and rewards GPs financially for achieving quality targets in areas that include BMI, waist circumference, HbA1c, blood pressure, total

Table 2.3 BLT T2D – Total Testosterone

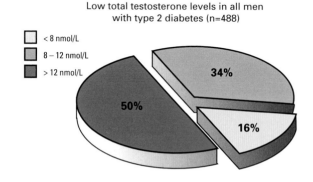

Low total testosterone levels in all men with type 2 diabetes (n=488)

- □ < 8 nmol/L
- ▨ 8 – 12 nmol/L
- ▩ > 12 nmol/L

Table 2.4 Free and total testosterone type 2 diabetic men - by decade

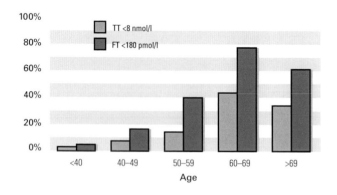

Table 2.5 BMI and waist circumference by total testosterone (nmol/L) in type 2 diabetes

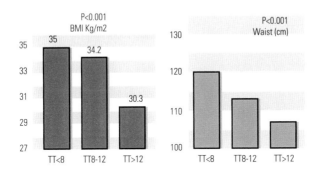

Table 2.6 ED (SHIM) associated with total (nmol/L) and free (pmol/L) testosterone in type 2 diabetes

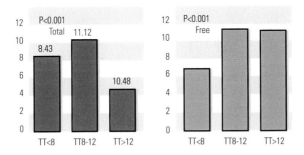

Table 2.7 HbA1c (%) and SHBG total testosterone (nmol/L) in type 2 diabetes

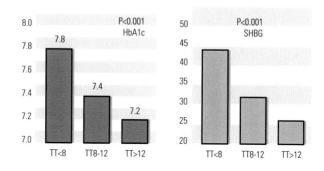

cholesterol, prescribing of ACE/ARBs, and eye and foot assessment. Results from the BLT study suggest strong associations with BMI, waist circumference and HbA1c. Patients with total and free testosterone in the lower tertiles had a mean BMI increase of 5, a waist circumference increase of 14cm and HbA1c of 7.81% v 7.20% compared with the upper tertile. Patients with TT and FT in the lower tertiles will not only be subject to the potentially greater risk associated with these levels but are significantly more likely to fall outside QOF (quality outcome framework) targets and result in underperformance. The current top HbA1c target of 7.5% is not being achieved by 50% of men in the low testosterone group versus 33% in the normal group. As this target is to be reduced to 7.0% for 2009/10[61] and possibly 6.5% in line with NICE guidance[62], these new targets may be very difficult to achieve with current strategies, particularly as conversion to insulin is associated with weight gain.

Original data from UKPDS (UK Prospective Diabetes Study)[63] showed that a 1% reduction in HbA1c was associated with 21% reduction in death, 14% reduction in myocardial infarction, 37% reduction in microvascular complications and 43% reduction in peripheral vascular disease, and recent 10-year follow up data[64] show that the benefits of tight control are maintained at 10 years. Recent data from the ADVANCE[65] study suggest a possible 10% reduction in macrovascular risk with a reduction to a target of 6.5% in conflict with data from the ACCORD study[66], which suggested possible risks with aggressive glucose lowering.

Currently, testosterone is not measured in UK and European diabetic practice. The usual reason stated in review articles[67] is the presumption that it is a consequence of the visceral obesity and ageing, or that the fall in SHBG associated with obesity in T2D will result in an adequate level of free testosterone. Published studies suggest that prevalence of testosterone deficiency is even greater if assessed by free testosterone[5,54,55,57]. Most cardiovascular risk factors are a consequence of ageing and yet routine multiple risk factors management in cardiovascular disease is standard practice in primary care, usually irrespective of age. Currently, diabetes care under the GP contract is target based. The workload is already onerous for clinicians, and routine questioning about ED and testosterone deficiency will lead to a considerable additional workload, without resources or remuneration.

When ED is detected, it will usually have to be managed, with associated prescribing cost and possible referral implications.

The prevalence of ED in the BLT study was 77% and was strongly associated with low free testosterone but not HbA1c, in contradiction to Romeo et al (*Table 2.8*) and Rhoden et al[68,69] who described a linear relationship with HbA1c in type 2 diabetics. This might be explained by the higher age group and greater associated co-morbidities in the BLT study group.

The three practices involved in the BLT study currently achieve maximum target QOF payments in diabetes and yet only 10% were currently taking ED therapy, and only 17% had ever taken medication[60]. NICE guidance on type 2 diabetes (May 2008)★ recommends that all men with diabetes are assessed annually for ED and offered full investigation and treatment with a PDE5 inhibitor. As ED prevalence is around 75%, current UK

Table 2.8 Glycaemic control correlates with ED

(*Romeo et al. J Urol 2000 163:788-7911*)

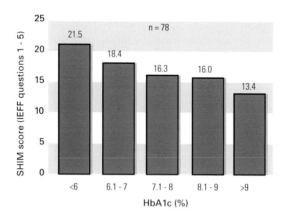

★ *NICE guidance 66 on Diabetes (May 2008) www.nice.org.uk/*

guidance[1] recommends that testosterone assessment in ED is mandatory, adherence to NICE guidance will necessitate frequent androgen testing in T2D. Based on recent evidence this will mean that a GP with a list size of 2,000 will have an estimated 40 men with T2D and 30 with ED and five with definite LOH with a TT of less than 8nmol/l. Currently this recommendation on ED is the only major item of NICE advice yet to be incorporated into the QOF. One interesting finding from this study was an initial reluctance by the trained diabetes nurses in the practices to administer the SHIM questionnaire in a face-to-face interview with the patient, insisting that the forms were sent out for postal return to the GP, reinforcing the view that embarrassment of healthcare professionals in discussing ED is still a significant problem.

The effects of testosterone replacement

The important question is whether restoration of testosterone to normal range will reduce risk and improve control. Two important questions need to be answered:

1. Can testosterone replacement improve the adverse biochemical profiles seen in T2D associated with low testosterone? Unfortunately, low testosterone is also associated with other cardiovascular disease which may be well established in this group.

2. Could treatment in the early stage of metabolic syndrome or glucose intolerance *prevent* progression to T2D and established CHD?

Interventional studies in T2D patients have shown a beneficial effect with testosterone therapy on insulin resistance. Kapoor et al[40] treated 24 patients with a short-acting testosterone injection (Sustanon®) every two weeks for a 12-week period. They found significant improvement in insulin resistance by homeostasis model assessment-insulin resistance (HOMA-1R) (-1.73), HbA1C (-0.37), and total cholesterol (-0.4%), but not blood pressure. The same authors also found beneficial effects on adipocytokines and C reactive protein levels[47].

Naharci et al[41] showed long-term benefit from testosterone supplementation on insulin resistance and visceral obesity, with improved results when levels were maintained in the upper rather than the low normal range.

Boyanov[42] et al investigated 48 middle-aged men with type 2 diabetes, (visceral) obesity and symptoms of androgen deficiency, in an open-label study. Twenty-four subjects received oral testosterone undecanoate (TU; 120 mg daily, for three months); 24 subjects received no treatment. Body composition was analysed by bio-impedance. Parameters of metabolic control were determined. Symptoms of androgen deficiency and erectile dysfunction were scored by self-administered questionnaires. TU had a positive effect on (visceral) obesity: statistically significant reduction in body weight (2.66%), waist-hip ratio (-3.96%) and body fat (-5.65%); negligible changes were found in the control group. TU significantly improved metabolic control: decrease in blood glucose values and mean HbA1c (from 10.4 to 8.6%).

TU treatment significantly improved symptoms of androgen deficiency (including erectile dysfunction), with virtually no change in the control group. There were no effects on blood pressure or haematological, biochemical and lipid parameters, and no adverse events.

In a small open label study of 32 men with metabolic syndrome, type 2 diabetes, and low free testosterone, Heufelder[70] found that transdermal testosterone Testogel®, Androgel® had an additional benefit compared with exercise and dietary advice alone. In cohort A (diet plus exercise) waist circumference fell from 107 to 102cm, HbA1c from 7.6 to 6.8%, triglycerides from 271 to 168% and HDL rose from 38 to 43mg/dL. In cohort B waist fell from 106 to 96, HbA1c from 7.5 to 6.3%, triglycerides from 285 to 149mg/dL, and HDL increased from 38 to 46mg/dL.

A multicentre randomised placebo controlled study of 2% transdermal testosterone gel (Tostran®, Tostrex®) in 220 men with metabolic syndrome and type 2 diabetes, the TIMES 2 study[71], showed significant improvement in insulin resistance, as assessed by the standard HOMA test, and HbA1c and symptom scores, particularly erectile function, at 12 months (*Tables 2.9, 2.10, 2.11*). This delayed response may explain the 50% discontinuation rate, which may prove a major drawback to this study. The findings also suggest that it may be up to 12 months for maximal improvement in HbA1c, although symptoms scores (particularly desire and ED) improve early. As the majority of patients in TIMES 2 had metabolic syndrome and not T2D, this suggests that in these cases a three-month trial may not be long enough to see metabolic benefits other than HOMA, which is not a standard assessment.

The BLT study forms the screening process for a double-blind placebo controlled intervention study of depot testosterone undecanoate 1,000mg in 200 patients, which commenced in October 2008 and will report in 2010.

TRT could be considered for a potential role in the treatment or prevention of metabolic syndrome. Until then, physicians must manage patients on best current evidence.[1, 72] Certainly the need to treat patients presenting with ED should enable the metabolic issues to be assessed on a case by case basis until firm guidance is available.

Larger studies on the metabolic effects of testosterone in T2D are being conducted to address the promising potential of metabolic benefits observed in these small studies. What is clear is that testosterone is an effective treatment for symptomatic testosterone deficiency and associated sexual dysfunctions, and that these symptoms are highly prevalent in the male T2D population.

Treating bothersome symptoms is likely to be appreciated by patients more than taking long-term medications on the basis of reducing statistical risk.

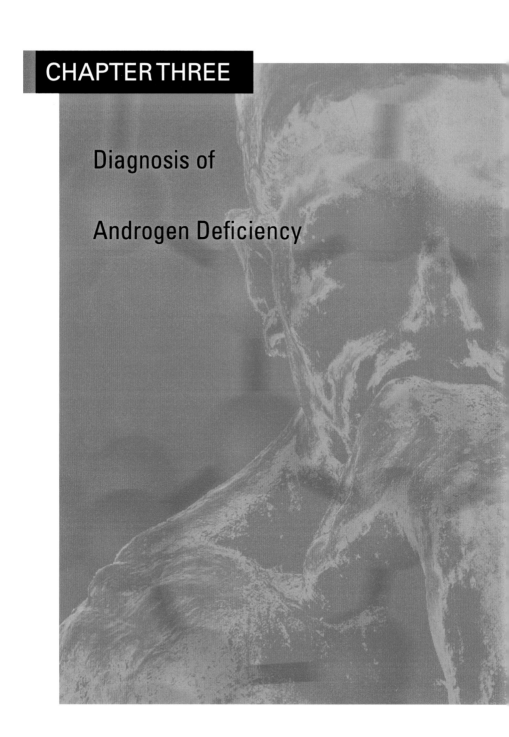

CHAPTER THREE

Diagnosis of

Androgen Deficiency

Diagnosis of androgen deficiency is based upon the identification of its non-specific features through clinical assessment and blood testing. As there is a diurnal variation in testosterone release, samples for testosterone assay should be drawn in the morning, between 08.00 and 11.00[1,72,73]. The assay should be repeated after two or three weeks, as testosterone is also released in a pulsatile manner and the result of a single assay may be misleading[8]. Men with a total serum testosterone (TT) that is consistently less than 12 nmol/L may benefit from testosterone replacement therapy and recent studies suggest that levels of up to 15 nmol/L are required for optimal sexual performance[41,53].

Current guidelines suggest that severe TDS is confirmed by a TT of less than 8 nmol/L or free testosterone less than 180 pmol/L. Borderline low TDS consists of TT 8-12 nmol/L or free testosterone 180-250 pmol/L. Free testosterone guidelines can be obtained by downloading the calculator from **www.issam.ch** and **www.HIM-link.com** or using the nomogram (*Appendix 1*), which assumes an albumin of 43 nmol/L. In reality, minor changes in albumin make little difference.

The symptoms and signs of hypogonadism are described in *Tables 3.1* and *3.2*

There is no evidence that giving testosterone to men with ED and normal androgen levels restores or improves their erectile function[1,72,73]. Hypogonadal men restored to the eugonadal state with testosterone replacement may experience a general improvement in sexual function, including erection;

Table 3.1 Androgen deficiency symptoms

Androgen deficiency symptoms	
Musculoskeletal	**Mood disorder and cognitive function**
Decreased vigour and physical energy	Irritability & lethargy
Diminished muscle strength	Decreased sense of well-being
Sexuality	Lack of motivation
Decreased interest in sex	Low mental energy
Reduction in frequency of sexual	Difficulty with short-term memory
activity	Depression
Poor erectile function/arousal	Low self-esteem
Loss of nocturnal erections	Insomnia
Reduced quality of orgasm	Nervousness
Reduced volume of ejaculate	**Vasomotor and nervous**
	Hot flushes
	Sweating

Table 3.2 Late onset hypogonadism physical signs

Late onset hypogonadism physical signs
Frequently, there are none
They may include
• Diminished muscle mass
• Loss of body hair
• Abdominal obesity
• Gynæcomastia
• Testes frequently normal, occasionally small

testosterone replacement therapy in this group might also restore or enhance responsiveness to PDE5 inhibitors[53]. Hypogonadism always has a cause and this cause should be established before treatment with testosterone is initiated. Traditionally[1,72,73], classification has been either:

1. **Primary**, due to failure of production by the testes, and usually associated with rises in LH and to a lesser extent FSH. Unfortunately in men over 50, this feedback response is blunted, mainly due to reduced receptor sensitivity and LH and FSH levels are usually within normal limits,

   or

2. **Secondary,** where LH and FSH levels are low due to a primary defect in the pituitary-hypothalamic axis, eg hyperprolactinaemia.

Rare causes of hypogonadism are described in *Table 3.3*[74]. With age, the feedback mechanism loses sensitivity, probably due to the pituitary ageing (*Table 3.4*) and reduced receptor sensitivity. In late onset hypogonadism, the LH and FSH are frequently normal. Prior assessment and safety monitoring should be performed according to contemporary authoritative guidelines[1, 72,73].

There is much debate as to whether we should be measuring free testosterone (FT), which constitutes around 2% of the total biologically available testosterone (BAT) (free and albumin bound), or the SHBG (sex hormone binding globulin), which

Table 3.3 Causes of hypogonadism

Causes of hypogonadism	
Primary congenital	**Secondary congenital**
Klinefelter's syndrome	Isolated GnRH deficiency
Noonan's syndrome	Isolated LH deficiency
Inborn errors of testosterone	Prader-Willi syndrome
biosynthesis	Laurence-Moon-Biedl syndrome
Androgen resistance states	
Primary acquired	**Secondary acquired**
Undescended testes	Pituitary tumours & infarct
Bilateral torsion of the testes	Trauma
Bilateral orchitis	Craniopharyngioma
Orchidectomy	Hyperprolactinaemia (1° & 2°)
Gonadal toxins (radiotherapy &	Haemochromatosis
chemotherapy)	Neurosarcoid
Acute and chronic systemic disease	Ageing

Table 3.4 Down-regulation in LOH

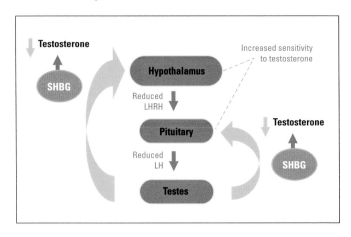

firmly binds testosterone to make it inactive. By calculating the total testosterone and SHBG, the free testosterone level can also be calculated using a formula found on **www.issam.ch** and **www.HIM-link.com**.[1,72,73]

Total testosterone is widely available for screening purposes and data from the HIM study[5] suggest that few cases will be missed

Figure 3.1 Age-related changes in serum concentrations of total and free testosterone, and sex hormone binding globulin[2]

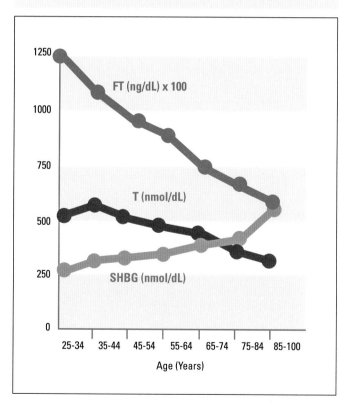

Diagnosis of Androgen Deficiency

if relying on at least two separate estimations plus clinical symptoms (*Table 3.2*)[40,1,72,73]. With age the SHBG rises and in diabetes and severe obesity, levels are lower[2]. In these cases more detailed bloods or endocrine opinion may be required.

For research and audit purposes the MASS questionnaire (*Appendix 3*) can be used. Copies can be obtained from **www.issam.ch** and **www.HIM-link.com**.

Practical issues for primary care

Patients are frequently diagnosed by screening tests for ED, as they usually want to know the cause of their loss of erections. When a low testosterone is detected, the anticipation would be that this abnormality will be corrected and that all will be well again. The patient will not be expecting the abnormality to be ignored and for potentially life long, expensive, on demand, self funded ED therapy. Testosterone replacement therapy (TRT) can be prescribed at NHS cost and may provide a number of possible additional benefits beyond improving erections, namely:

1. Improving sexual desire (often diminished in ageing men with ED)

2. Improving ejaculatory and orgasmic function

3. Possible improvement in well-being, cognitive function, depression and quality of life.

From the couple's perspective, it is important that TRT would permit these improvements without the limitations of on demand therapy restricted to once per week.

Evidence suggests that around 10% of ED cases may be associated with low testosterone and that improvements of 60% could be expected when it is the sole abnormality. More usually, there are associated vascular or relationship factors and this response rate with TRT alone is more like 30%[1]. This is still significant and should be negotiated with couples on an individual basis. A three-month trial of TRT is reasonable in such cases, explaining to the patient that additional treatment may be required. A treatment algorithm has been suggested in Standard Practice in Sexual Medicine[74].

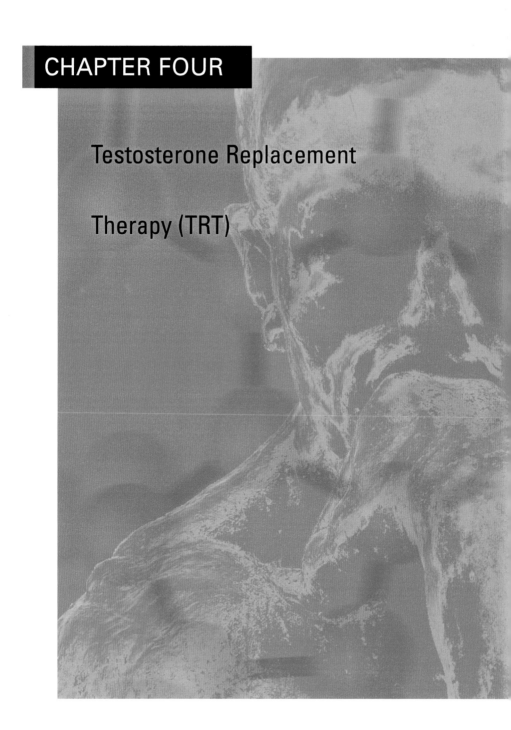

CHAPTER FOUR

Testosterone Replacement

Therapy (TRT)

Current published guidance from the BSSM, European Urology Association and the International Society for the Ageing Male[1,72,73] suggests treatment at the following levels:

Normal:	TT >12 nmol/L TRT not normally required
Grey Zone:	TT 12–8 nmol/L – consider three-month T trial
Testosterone Deficiency Syndrome:	TT <8 nmol/L (231 ng/L) = supplementation

A range of well-tolerated testosterone presentations are available:

1. Oral therapies may aid compliance but are generally not recommended due to the possible hepatic toxicity and the need for frequent dosing.[1,72,73] A buccal formulation avoids hepatic risks, but this has not proved popular to date.

2. Long-acting (three-monthly) testosterone injection of testosterone undecanoate has advantages over the older less expensive fortnightly or monthly injections as they produce more consistent levels of testosterone resulting in fewer mood swings[75].

3. Daily (morning) application of a transdermal testosterone gel is acceptable to most men[76].
   Patches are also effective but currently these are large

and can be conspicuous, with skin reactions in around 28% of cases[77].

4. Testosterone implants were once popular but infection, extrusion and tachyphylaxis have proved problematical. Implants are inexpensive but require a 2-3 monthly minor operative procedure.[1,73]

The common indication for testosterone therapy is the finding of a low or low/normal testosterone level in patients presenting with erectile dysfunction, and the current recommended algorithms for managing patients with and without ED are shown below (*Figure 4.1*). Most endocrinologists would suggest treating men with testosterone below 8 nmol/L but much higher levels are required for optimal sexual response to PDE5i and a landmark study by Shabsigh[41] et al demonstrated the potential for salvaging patients by restoring low or borderline testosterone to levels of around 14 nmol/L or above.

Current opinion is that testosterone should be restored to the upper physiological levels first as approximately 30% of cases of ED[41] will be corrected by this alone, especially in patients without other significant risk factors. Such an approach is logical and cost effective, especially as licensed therapies for ED usually have to be funded by the patient.

Long-term monitoring

Although there is no evidence from over 60 years of clinical use of testosterone that TRT causes cancer[78] or BPH (benign prostatic hypertrophy)[79], it is generally accepted that it may

Figure 4.1 Treatment algorithm for androgen therapy in patients presenting with ED[1, 72, 73]

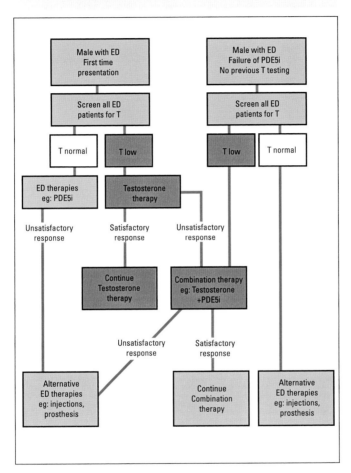

exacerbate an existing prostate cancer. The consensus of opinion is that it is wise to monitor elderly patients on TRT. The background prevalence of Ca prostate is around 0.55% per annum and there is evidence that elderly men may harbour

Testosterone Replacement Therapy (TRT)

pre-cancerous lesions of neoplasia (PIN) that would be missed by reliance on PSA (prostate specific antigen) and DRE (digital rectal examination)[80] (*see Table 4.1*).

Table 4.1 Occult prostate cancer in hypogonadal men[82]

77 men (mean age 58 years)
TT <10.4 nmol/l
PSA ≤ 3.9 and DRE – ve
Sextant biopsy
• 14% prostate cancer plus 8.1% PIN 3
• 29% men ≥ 60 years had cancer

The concern is that an undiagnosed occult focus could be activated by testosterone therapy. Prostate cancer, particularly more aggressive forms, is actually more common in hypogonadal men[81] and prostate cancer rates rise as testosterone levels fall with age (*Figure 4.2*).

Figure 4.2 Incidence of prostate cancer and total testosterone[83]

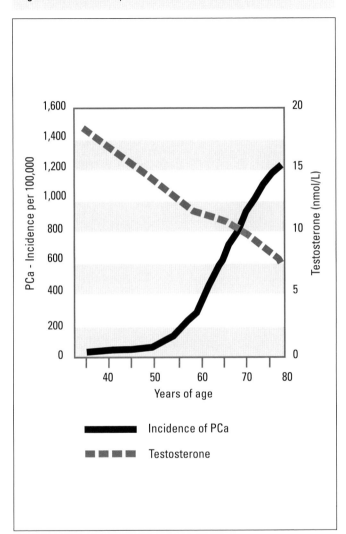

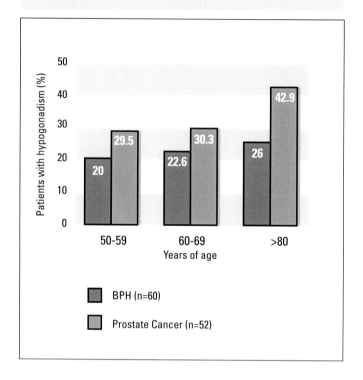

Figure 4.3 Hypogonadism in men with BPH vs. men with prostate cancer
(Schatzl G et al, 2001 & 2003) [83,84]

Schatzl[83,84] evaluated cohorts of men with BPH and those with prostate cancer and found higher rates of hypogonadism in the cancer group. Two large reviews[85,86], have shown that patients presenting with more invasive prostate cancers (Gleason score >8) tend to have lower testosterone (*Figure 4.3*) and suggests that that low testosterone might be an independent predictor for extra-prostatic spread.

A recent review of published studies on testosterone therapy

Figure 4.4 Testosterone therapy and the development of prostate cancer

(Hoffman MA , DeWolf WC, Morgentaler A: Is low serum free testosterone a marker for high grade prostate cancer? J Urol 2000; 163: 824-7)

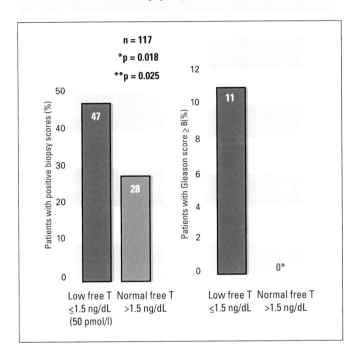

and subsequent prostate cancer also produced reassuring data, with a mean prostate cancer rate of 1%, which is similar to screening studies[87,88,89] (*Table 4.2*). Many studies used older regimes, involving oral therapy or shorter acting injection. Modern transdermal or depot injection should be considered for longer term use as they may produce fewer peaks and troughs and a corresponding more favourable safety profile.

Testosterone Replacement Therapy (TRT)

Table 4.2 PCa during testosterone therapy

	ART (months)	Patients	PCa
Hajjar, 1997	24	45	–
Sih, 1997	12	17	–
Dobs, 1999	24	66	3
Snyder, 1999	36	54	1
Snyder, 2000	36	18	0
Wang, 2000	6	76	0
Kenny, 2001	12	34	0
Wang, 2004	36	123	3
TOTAL		**433**	**7 (1.6%)**

However, there are limitations to published follow-up studies of testosterone therapy, such as:

◆ Small sample sizes

◆ Selection bias

◆ Short follow-up period, while prostate cancer is a slow-growing tumour

◆ Mainly epidemiological observations with historical correlations on risk

◆ No randomisation according to baseline levels, thus:

• increased possibility that many patients were eugonadal vs. hypogonadal

• the effect of testosterone substitution on prostate cancer risk is still not known in eugonadal men.

A few small studies have suggested no increase in PSA levels or reactivation of disease in patients successfully treated with testosterone after radical prostatectomy[90] but such cases need to be evaluated on an individual basis.

Shabsigh[89] et al recently reviewed 197 papers and articles on testosterone therapy and concluded once again that there was no evidence to associate testosterone therapy with any increased risk of prostate cancer. There are probable benefits for men on testosterone therapy receiving regular monitoring where there is no national screening policy for the early detection of prostate cancer. Perhaps the time has come to finally reassure patients. For too long this over-cautious approach has prevented patients from receiving effective treatments for bothersome symptoms and delayed important research into diabetes and cardiovascular disease.

Hyperprolactinaemia (HPL)

HPL is associated with ED, loss of sexual interest and anorgasmia. It is frequently accompanied by androgen deficiency, as high prolactin levels suppress LH production and, consequently, cause hypogonadism. Hyperprolactinaemia should be excluded by blood testing in all men with reduced sexual interest. Moderate elevation of prolactin levels (<1000 mIU/L) is unlikely to cause ED[91]. HPL is found in 1-2% of ED patients; a third of these will be due to pituitary adenomas.

It is common practice to check the prolactin level if a low testosterone is found, usually at the stage of rechecking the testosterone level. This is cost effective but significant hyperprolactinaemia is rarely found with a normal testosterone.

Hyperprolactinaemia may be due to stress and drugs (notably metoclopramide, chlorpromazine, and several other antipsychotics[92]). A small proportion of men with hyperprolactinaemia will be found to have a prolactin-secreting pituitary tumour, but these must not be missed. Hyperprolactinaemia is common in men on dialysis for chronic renal failure. Unless an obvious cause is found and the prolactin levels return to normal, referral to an endocrinologist is advisable.

Between 10-22% of patients with HPL[93] will have macro-hyperprolactinaemia, a biologically inactive variant, which can be detected on immunoassay. These patients are usually well but still need CT scanning to exclude adenoma; they do not usually respond to prolactin lowering drugs.

Treatment of ED associated with HPL should be focused on treatment of the cause of the raised prolactin to reduce the levels. Bromocriptine daily or cabergolide[94] weekly will restore erections in around two-thirds of patients, with improvement of sexual desire and well-being. Patients with macro-adenomas on CT scan should be referred to an ophthalmologist or neurosurgeon.

Thyroid disease

Hyper- and hypothyroidism may influence erectile function by increasing SHBG production, thereby reducing FT levels. Effective treatment of hyperthyroidism may resolve coexisting ED. Provided that there is no other contraindication, ED treatment may be provided until the patient is rendered euthyroid through other treatments[1].

Current guidance on testosterone therapy

Current EAU, ISSAM and BSSM[1,79,80] guidance is that patients should have a prostate assessment by baseline PSA (plus ideally DRE) with follow-up within three months and then annually. This should be accompanied by a morning total or free testosterone (if locally available), plus an annual full blood count.

The timing of blood tests (pre 11am) is more important in the monitoring of patients on transdermal preparations rather than depot of implants. The aim is to maintain patients in the upper range of normal and this will frequently require a dose greater than 50mg per day (average 75mg). This may have cost implications as the price of testosterone gels may double if a second sachet is required. In the case of long-acting depot injections, the usual advice is to reduce the interval between injections by two weeks, which has less cost implication.

Hypogonadal men usually have smaller prostates with lower PSAs, and TRT results in a restoration of PSA to 'normal levels' within the first six months. Rises outside the normal range would suggest the possibility that the patient might have an occult focus of malignancy and should be referred.[79,80]

It should be emphasised that there is no evidence from several metanalyses that restoration of normal testosterone levels with TRT is associated with a risk of prostate malignancy[89] or BPH.

One of the issues is that whilst the benefits of TRT in terms of sexual function, well-being, metabolic and cardiovascular disease will be appreciated by physicians, the burden of prostate vigilance will fall upon under-resourced urologists.

Adverse events

Irritation of the skin, related to adhesive, occurs in 2%[77,78] of men on patches. Some patients dislike the smell of gels and it is recommended that they apply these in the morning to either the shoulders or upper arms, or in the case of the 2% gel formulation to the inner thighs and abdomen. Occasionally minimal transmission to the partner occurs if the gel is used at night. Few men complain of hirsuitism, voice change or greasy skin, and hair loss is very rare. Injectable testosterone formulations are associated with injection pain in about 10% of patients. Liver problems are not seen with modern formulations and monitoring is not required. Known prostate cancer is an absolute contraindication. For patients on anticoagulation, minor dose adjustments are rarely required.

The current situation in relation to testosterone therapy is unclear but the bulk of evidence suggests that therapy is associated with a favourable safety profile and that some men will benefit from treatment. Long-term clinical trials are needed but the methodology of such trials is complex and, for economical reasons, many well not be conducted.

As physicians with a specialist interest, we are faced with patients who would like to know what we believe to be the most appropriate therapy for them now, in the light of our current knowledge. It is our duty as clinicians to give them the advice that we perceive is in their best interests, assessing their priorities. Whereas long-term studies are desirable to fully evaluate many of the issues described in earlier chapters, particularly in relation to diabetes, it is important to realise that testosterone is fully licensed as a treatment for hypogonadism and testosterone deficiency syndrome (TDS), irrespective of whether other benefits might result. Many men are experiencing bothersome symptoms which bring them to their doctor. Modern primary care has probably become too orientated towards the management of statistical risk but we should not apologise for improving patients' symptoms and quality of life. The patient might not be alive when the results of the perfect RCT become available!

The Role of Androgens in Men's Health

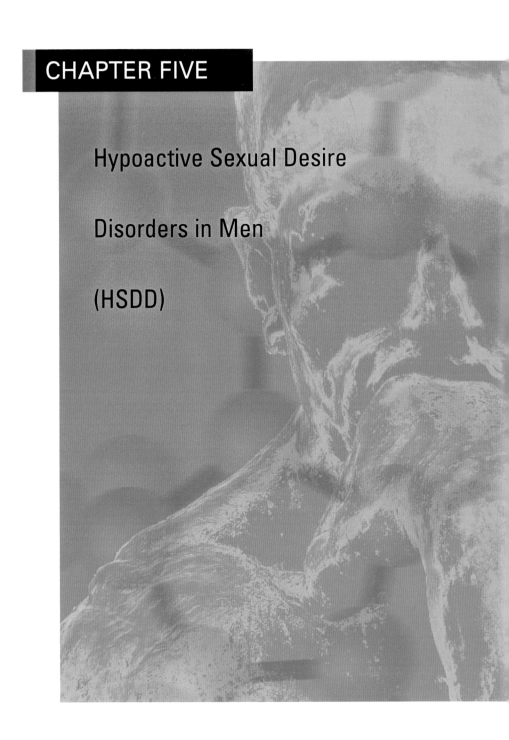

CHAPTER FIVE

Hypoactive Sexual Desire

Disorders in Men

(HSDD)

Introduction

HSDD was recognized as a clinical entity in 1977 and defined in DSM IV as:

> *"Persistently or recurrently deficient (or absent) sexual fantasy or desire for sexual activity, leading to marked distress or interpersonal difficulty, unless explained by another medical disorder."*[95]

Desire is defined as *"the motivation or inclination to be sexual"*.

Kaplan's model[96] of the male sexual response concludes that desire in men is innate and spontaneous, leading to arousal, comprising erection and excitement, leading to orgasm and detumescence.

Levine[97] has suggested that desire should be considered in terms of:

- **Drive,** which is the biological component of desire. This might one day be described in terms of neurophysiology (*Tables 1 and 2*)

- **Motive,** which is individual and related to relationship psychology. This could be considered in terms of "she might leave me unless I have sex with her". The motivational component is probably more pronounced in female desire

- **Wish,** the cultural component. This can be considered in terms of what the culture regards as a "true man".

HSDD frequently co-exists with other sexual disorders[98], particularly erectile dysfunction, and the management of the combined conditions often requires specific clinical decisions and actions[99].

Epidemiology

The 1992 National Health and Social Life Survey[100] reviewed 1,410 men aged 18-59 in the US. They reported a prevalence of 5% HSDD compared with 5% for erectile dysfunction. The prevalence of desire disorders in the female cohort was 23%.

More recently, the Global Sexual Attitudes and Behaviours Study (GSSAB)[101], an international survey of 13,618 men from 29 countries, included the single question as to whether lack of sexual interest occurred occasionally, periodically or frequently, with ranges between 28% and 12.5%. Older age, depression, high alcohol consumption, emotional problems or stress and poor general health were the major risk factors.

Predictors of low desire (with odds ratios) were:

- ◆ Thinking about sex less than once per week: **3.63**
- ◆ Any same sex activity ever: **2.51**
- ◆ Partner ever had abortion: **1.98**
- ◆ Sexually "touched" before puberty: **2.23**

Table 5.1 Sources of desire

Desire sources
• Desire centre in limbic system of the brain
• Desire modulated by inhibitors and enhancers:
– Hormonal factors – testosterone
– Physical factors
– Cognitive/ emotional factors
– Relationship factors

Table 5.2 Components of male sexual desire

Male sexual drive is described as:
• More urgent
• Less distractible
• More goal focused
• More focused on intercourse and orgasm

Table 5.3 Assessing sexual desire

Always/usually/sometimes/never
• Pleasurable thoughts about sex?
• Do you initiate lovemaking?
• Easy to get and stay aroused?
• Sexual fantasies?
• Responsive to partner's overtures?
• Self stimulation?
• Do you miss sex?

Physiology of desire and drive disorders in men

Androgens[102] are the major hormones regulating the biologic component of desire. Table 4 summarises the sources and relative potencies. Oestrogen, progesterone, oxytocin and prolactin have negative effects[102] and the role of alcohol as an inhibitor of desire is predominantly by central effects and by inducing hepatic conversion of testosterone to oestrogen. Cortisol has a negative effect on desire, seen in Cushing's syndrome. Cutler[103] showed the importance of pheromones in sexual desire in men and women, the potency of which has not escaped the perfume industry.

Serotonin usually has a negative effect, predominantly associated with feedback from interference with arousal and orgasm, as seen with most non-selective SSRIs[104]. Dopamine, agonists, particularly Apomorphine, and L-Dopa derivatives, have been associated with increased desire, occasionally a problem in elderly male patients with Parkinson's disease. Histamine is thought to have a negative effect on desire. The H2 receptor blockers, cimetidine and ranitidine, are associated with erectile dysfunction and oestrogenic properties, particularly gynaecomastia[105]. Moderate levels of hyper-thyroidism[47] can enhance desire, whereas hypothyroidism is associated with reduced desire in men and women.

Table 5.4 Relative potency of androgens

Sources and relative potencies of androgens	
DHT (dihydrotestosterone)	300
Testosterone	100
Androstenedione (adrenal)	10
DHEA, DHEA-S (adrenal)	5

Desire and relationship dynamics

Kaplan's model[96] for male and female desire describes inciting factors activating the hypothalamic and limbic sex regulating centres and suppressing factors in desire, such as hormones, drugs and depression, along with inhibitors such as unattractive partners, negative thoughts, anti-fantasies, negative emotions, stress and anger. A frequent response to lack of desire is sexual avoidance. This may be associated with primary lack of desire or secondary to an associated disorder, particularly ED or PE (premature ejaculation). Such issues can disturb the dynamics of the relationship as desire disorders are more common in women, and low desire in the partner can create a desire disparity where the partner feels a pressure to become the initiator as she feels that the relationship might be threatened if intercourse is not taking place. In some relationships the partner with the lower desire, particularly associated with sexual avoidance, holds the balance of power, and frequently uses this against the partner as a way of punishment or dealing with hostility towards them.

Hypoactive Sexual Desire Disorders in Men (HSDD)

Clinical evaluation of desire disorders

Frequently cases present with an associated ED or PE and specific questions should be directed towards[105]:

- Sexual frequency (although sometimes frequency is normal but without desire)

- Sexual thoughts

- Sexual fantasies

- Initiation of sexual activity and changes (*see Table 5.3*).

Investigations include fasting glucose, lipids, morning testosterone, LH and thyroid function tests. Corona et al reported some element of HSSD in 43% of 428 men with ED[106].

Management

Many patients do not suffer distress and do not wish treatment, particularly if there is no disparity with their partner. Frequently the higher desire female partner demands action as *"Men should not be like this,"* in effect they do not fit the conventional stereotype.

TRT can be effective (see Chapter 3) where there is evidence of hypogonadism; likewise, correction of hypothyroidism may be beneficial. Co-incidental ED should be treated as in *Chapter 2*.

The treatment of associate depression[104] can be beneficial, particularly if SSRIs with higher rates of sexual dysfunction are avoided. Mirtazepine[107] may be the antidepressant with the best profile in such cases. Bupropion has been used with success in HSSD in the US and two trials reported good results, mainly in women. Bupropion[108] has been used mainly for smoking cessation in the UK, and reported side effects and the lack of a licensed indication will preclude the use in HSSD.

A novel serotonin modulator, a 5HT1A agonist and 5HT2A antagonist, flibanserin, is being developed to treat HSDD in women with eventual plans for treatment in men. There may be more ethical concerns in the use of centrally acting drugs to treat HSDD in men than women.[109]

Relationship therapy, either alone or combined with the above,[110] is frequently required. Specific psychotherapy usually has the following components:

- Affectual awareness to address the sources of negative and positive emotions
- Insight and understanding
- Cognitive and systemic therapy
- Behavioural intervention

It is unlikely that the primary care physician will be able to deliver the full range of therapy without the need for specialist support.

Hypoactive Sexual Desire Disorders in Men (HSDD)

Conclusions

Hypoactive sexual desire disorders in men are under-diagnosed and frequently labelled as erectile dysfunction, which may be a frequent primary or secondary association. Such patients often respond poorly to ED therapy and infrequent attempts with prescribed medication are an important pointer to HSDD.

A significant cause for under-diagnosis is the myth that all men innately possess sexual desire and that low desire is almost exclusively a condition of women. There has been an understandable lack of development of new pharmaceutical products to treat low desire in men, possibly for fear of litigation issues involving possible allegations of rape or abuse. Testosterone is currently the only licensed therapy to treat HSDD in men and has recently been licensed in low dose patch formulation to treat HSDD in surgically postmenopausal women as Intrinsa®![10]

Depression and psychotropic medication are common causes and appropriate prescribing by physicians may reduce the impact of HSDD on patients. The impact of poorly diagnosed and treated HSDD on the relationship is considerable.

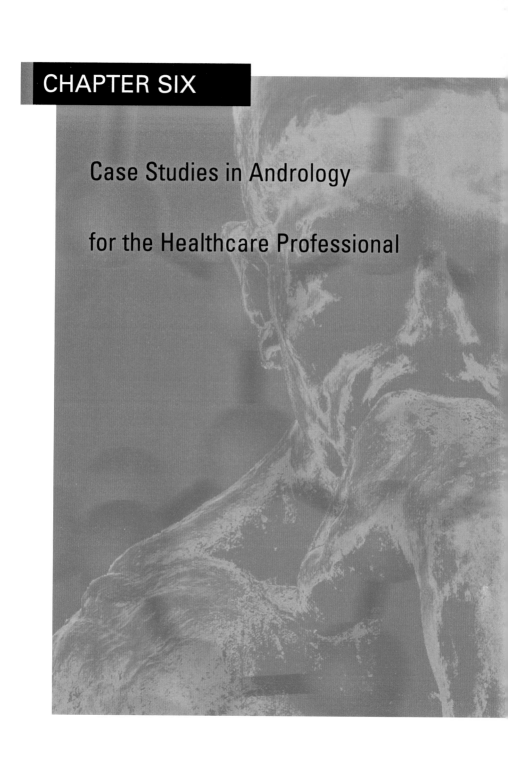

CHAPTER SIX

Case Studies in Andrology

for the Healthcare Professional

Introduction

Sexual problems are essentially about couples and relationships, and the following case histories from the author's clinical practice should reinforce many of the learning points from the earlier chapters. Most healthcare professionals receive little undergraduate or postgraduate education in sexual medicine and the following cases may be useful as tutorials for students and registrars.

Case study 1

David is a 63 year old man married to Dawn (45) for three years, a second marriage following the death of his first wife. He is hypertensive on valsarten, felodipine and doxazacin, and simvastatin, with finasteride 5mg for well controlled BPH. His PSAs have been elevated (between 4.0 and 6.5) over the past three years but four biopsies have shown only BPH. Since commencing finasteride, his BPH has fallen to 3.1. He expresses a reluctance to undergo further biopsies.

He presents with erectile dysfunction, which has been getting worse for five years with no morning erections. Initially Dawn was understanding, but David now feels that his relationship is threatened. He feels less interested in sex, more tired than usual. His GP gave him eight doses of sildenafil 100mg with only partial response. Vardenafil 20mg gave a similar response.

Case Studies in Andrology for the Healthcare Professional

Bloods results – cholesterol 4.5, fasting glucose 4.8 and total testosterone of 9.5 nmol/L. Repeat testosterone was 8.8 and prolactin 125 nmol/l.

After considerable discussion, he is commenced on testosterone gel 50mg/5g daily and notices improvement in his sexual desire and well-being, but only has partial erections. Tadalafil 20mg is added and he reports that by taking 20mg on Friday and Tuesday evenings, he and Dawn are enjoying intercourse four times per week as they have years of catching up to do!

After six months he visits his urologist and his PSA has risen to 4.5 and it is suggested that he stops his testosterone. After three months he returns with loss of erections, once again requesting to restart testosterone.

Key learning points

- There are frequently multiple pathologies in ageing males
- The efficacy of PDE5 inhibitors is enhanced by correction of borderline testosterone levels
- Testosterone has additional benefits in sexual function other than improvement of ED
- Finasteride therapy is associated with a drop of approximately 50% in PSA. Testosterone therapy is associated with transient increases in PSA
- Improvement in sexual function is greatly valued by many patients, even if there is perceived to be a potential health risk.

Case study 2

Frank is 58 and presents with complete loss of erections and avoidance of sexual intercourse with his wife Ruby over the past three years. He suffers from type 2 diabetes and hypertension and takes metformin, perindopril and simvastatin. He was commenced on sildenafil 100mg with no response.

Blood tests: glucose 8.0, cholesterol 3.8, morning testosterone 4.5 nmol/L (repeat 6.2), PSA 1.5.

He was commenced on sustanon injections 250mg every four weeks with no response after three months. A serum prolactin was 1200 and he is referred for CT scan, which reveals a small pituitary adenoma. Treatment with bromocriptine results in improvement in erections after three months, but sildenafil 100mg is still required for full erection.

Key learning points

■ Hyperprolactinaemia is a rare cause of ED, is usually associated with low testosterone levels, and sometimes only diagnosed after failure to respond to testosterone

■ Multiple pathologies may exist in the same patient and may dictate that each condition is treated. The most common cause of hyperprolactinaemia is a micro adenoma of the pituitary gland.

Case study 3

Albert is 73 and was diagnosed with prostate cancer five years ago and successfully treated with a non-nerve sparing radical prostatectomy. He developed erectile dysfunction after the operation and has failed to respond to all three PDE5 inhibitors, MUSE and alprostadil injections. He has suffered with depression for three years and takes citalopram 40mg daily. Examination reveals a large plaque of dorsal Peyronie's disease.

Blood tests reveal cholesterol of 7.5, fasting glucose 6.9 mmol/L and morning testosterone of 4.5 nmol/L. PSA is 0.2.

He is commenced on testosterone gel, but after three months there is no improvement in erections and he is switched to depot testosterone undecanoate 1,000 mg, repeated after six weeks. With the help of caverject 20mcg he is able to maintain an erection for penetration. He notices a significant improvement in mood.

Repeat testosterone after six months has risen to 10.4 nmol/l, fasting glucose 4.2, cholesterol 6.2 and PSA 1.0.

■ Multiple pathologies may co-exist in ageing males

■ Successful radical prostatectomy is associated with a high risk of ED and does not preclude physiological doses of testosterone. Some patients may be resistant to transdermal testosterone but respond to injections

■ Specific ED therapy may still be required and oral PDE5 inhibitors only work in around 35% of post radical prostatectomy patients

■ Testosterone therapy may improve glucose tolerance and symptoms of depression

■ Peyronie's disease does not usually require treatment when angulation still allows penetration, usually above 45 degrees.

Case study 4

Steve and Diane have been married for nine months. It is the second marriage for both. Steve's wife left him for a work colleague after a long affair and Diane left her alcoholic husband. She had no children and Steve's two children are with his first wife. It is noticeable that Diane does most of the talking throughout. The complaint is that he never initiates intercourse since they were married, and when they do make love, he cannot maintain his erection. He never masturbates, gets few spontaneous erections and never gets sexual fantasies. His investigations are as follows:

Case Studies in Andrology for the Healthcare Professional

Fasting glucose	4.2
Cholesterol	5.9
Testosterone	12.2

He was started on sildenafil 50mg and reviewed at six weeks. He has only taken one tablet as he has been working away from home a lot. He says that he finds it "artificial". He is switched to tadalafil 20mg and instructed to take it twice weekly on a regular basis, once again returning six weeks later with one failed attempt. On this occasion, he attends without Diane, admitting that he finds Diane unattractive as she has put on a lot of weight since the marriage (he weighs 130kg!). He has begun seeing another woman whilst working away from home in London and is having no problem with erections.

You recommend relationship therapy but learn six months later that they have split up.

Key learning points

- HSDD frequently presents as another dysfunction, particularly ED
- Patients and their partners may manipulate the consultation to avoid facing the real issues
- Relationship issues are common with HSDD
- The medical treatment of HSDD is disappointing
- Often, despite our best attempts, relationships will fail.

Case 5

Peter is 54 and a successful company director. He suffers from mild hypertension and takes lisinopril 5mg daily. He complains of total lack of interest in sex for the last three years and gets few spontaneous erections. He blames his lifestyle, with frequent international travel and evening meetings. He rarely takes a holiday and his wife, Liz (52), has also lost interest in sex since her hysterectomy five years ago. They have drifted apart and feel that they are now just friends. Liz went to relationship therapy but Peter was too busy to attend.

On direct questioning, it becomes clear that Peter experienced a couple of episodes of ED over three years ago when Liz reluctantly agreed to intercourse not long after her hysterectomy. Around this time, Liz never initiated sex, whereas previously she had been the main initiator. His blood tests show well controlled BP and cholesterol, normal fasting glucose and testosterone 11.0 nmol/L.

You initiate treatment with tadalafil 20mg on demand, but he only takes one tablet and returns four weeks later to say that it did not work. You ask why he did not try more and he states that they have both been busy with work and their daughter's wedding. You add testosterone gel 50mg daily for two weeks and tell him to take tadalafil regularly every Friday and Tuesday, and have intercourse when he feels in

Case Studies in Andrology for the Healthcare Professional

the mood. You explain to both of them that hypertension can be associated with ED and that low or borderline testosterone can be associated with sub-optimal response to therapy. You also explain that relationship problems frequently occur secondary to this, and that they need to communicate more rather than use excuses.

You see them after two months and they have managed intercourse three times with total spontaneity and booked a holiday together. Liz has seen her GP and commenced HRT.

Key learning points

■ HSDD is frequently secondary to a change in sexual desire in the partner, creating a 'desire disparity'

■ Successful men frequently deal with sexual failure by withdrawing contact, rather than confronting the issue

■ Low desire in a partner, ED and borderline testosterone often co-exist and focusing on one problem as 'the cause' can be unhelpful

■ A strategy that works is the most important goal, and this may involve combining medications for both partners, as well as relationship therapy.

Case study 6

Michael is 46 and divorced from Jane seven years ago. They had two children but Jane could not take the pill, blaming weight gain and depression. Michael had a vasectomy but they split up six months later. Four years ago Michael met Debbie, 35, a successful lawyer, keen to have children. Michael paid to have his vasectomy reversed and they are on their third course of private IVF. Michael and Debbie attend as he complains that he is too tired and busy and sexual attempts are taking place less than once a week.

In private, John admits that he is avoiding sexual contact as he finds sex has become a chore and all Debbie talks about is the IVF programme. He says that he still loves her but is uncertain about the future. All his investigations are normal and his testosterone is 27 nmol/L

You recommend private referral to an experienced sex therapist. You find out later that they have abandoned the IVF programme. They state that they are both happier since making the decision!

Key learning points

■ Problems with female contraception are often a reason for deciding upon vasectomy

■ Vasectomy is associated with an increased risk of relationship breakdown and requests for reversal are increasing

■ Infertility issues can be strongly associated with decline in male sexual desire

■ Desire problems in the male are often neglected by couples undergoing infertility treatments

■ Relationship and sex therapy should be considered routinely in such cases.

Case study 7

Frank, a 62 year old long distance lorry driver, was involved in a fatal crash when his lorry jack-knifed on a frozen road late at night. The driver of an oncoming vehicle was killed, but Frank escaped with only cuts and grazes. For four weeks he was unable to sleep but went back to work after only a couple of days, as he felt that was the best way of dealing with his problem. For the next two months he experienced outbursts of temper, poor sleep, with flashbacks of the accident, and on several occasions had to pull the car over because he was shaking and light headed. His wife suggested that he saw his GP, who prescribed fluoxetine 20mg. He returned after three weeks and was increased to 40mg with some improvement.

Twelve months after the accident, he returned to see his GP with loss of erections and was prescribed 50mg of sildenafil privately (four tablets) but returned three months later saying that it had not worked. He and his wife June had always enjoyed a very active sex life right up until the accident. His insurance company had arranged a referral to a private urologist to assess the relevance of the accident and subsequent depression, and its association with his ED. The urologist reported that organic ED could not have been caused by his injuries and diagnosed 'psychogenic' ED, suggesting that he be referred for sex therapy. Frank requested a second opinion as the case was shortly going to court and he was claiming £30,000 for ED as a consequence of his accident.

At second opinion, the author confirmed that he was in fact suffering from hypoactive sexual desire disorder, secondary to post-traumatic stress disorder. In fact, he had made no sexual attempts since the accident, avoided all possible sexual contact with June and increased his workload to be away from home more often. He took two doses of sildenafil 50mg, without telling June, and sat in a chair without any sexual stimulation. His sexual desire was virtually non-existent from the time of starting fluoxetine.

Key learning points

■ A full sexual history would have elicited the lack of sexual attempts and stimulation

■ Do not believe the patient's opinion of their problem

■ HSDD is often associated with post-traumatic stress and he would have grounds for compensation as part of his claim

■ This patient should have been given a full ED assessment for cardiovascular risk, diabetes, hypogonadism and dyslipidaemia, despite the history. The GP did not put himself in a position to diagnose the patient correctly

■ The GP may be liable for not assessing the case and not warning about the possible sexual side-effects of the fluoxetine.

Discontinuation of fluoxetine and relationship therapy improved the problem. He was found to have mild type 2 diabetes and his erections improved with tadalafil 20mg twice weekly under the severe distress regime. His testosterone and lipids were normal.

Case study 8

Rashid is a 55 year old consultant psychiatrist who presented to his GP three years ago with depressive symptoms. He was a moderately controlled type 2 diabetic, and at the time he was working hard due to staff shortages. His GP referred him to a consultant colleague at his own hospital. He was advised to take time from work and was treated with three different SSRI antidepressants over six months and was eventually advised to take early retirement on grounds of stress. Six months later, he consulted his GP with ED (which he had experienced for three years) and loss of libido. His GP tried sildenafil 50mg with no response and referred him to the ED clinic.

Routine bloods in the clinic revealed a total testosterone of 5.5 nmol/L, SHBG 24 nmol/L and free testosterone 140 pmol/L. He was treated with tadalafil 20mg thrice weekly and testosterone gel 75mg per day, and improved dramatically. He returned after four months with a total testosterone of 13.0, SHBG 38 and free testosterone 240. He felt better than for several years but unfortunately he no longer had a consultant post. Two months later a consultant colleague had to retire early on health grounds and Rashid returned to full time locum consultant work. He commented on how many patients with similar symptoms he might have misdiagnosed.

Key learning points

■ A full sexual history would have elicited the lack of sexual attempts and stimulation

■ Hypogonadism is commonly associated with T2D

■ Symptoms of testosterone deficiency are commonly misdiagnosed as depression

■ Patients frequently do not mention ED or loss of libido unless asked directly, especially professional colleagues

■ Testosterone should be measured in ALL cases of ED

■ Testosterone deficiency should be suspected in all older depressed patients who fail to respond to antidepressant therapy.

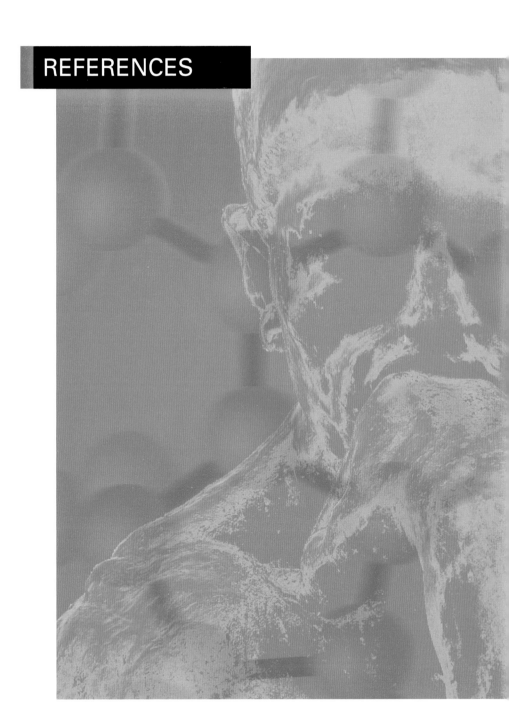

REFERENCES

References

1. Hackett G, Kell P, Ralph D et al. British Society for Sexual Medicine Guidelines on the Management of Erectile Dysfunction. *J Sex Med* 2008;5:8 1841-1846

2. Morley JE, Kaiser FE, Perry HM 3rd, Patrick P, Morley PM, Stauber PM, Vellas B, Baumgartner RN, Garry PJ. Longitudinal changes in testosterone, luteinizing hormone, and follicle-stimulating hormone in healthy older men. *Metabolism.* 1997 Apr;46(4):410-3

3. White A. Life expectancy in European Men and Women *JMHG* Vol1 2004. 5-8

4. Araujo AB, Durante R, Feldman HA. The relationship between depressive symptoms and male erectile dysfunction: cross sectional results from the MMAS. *Psycosom med* 1998; 60: 458-465

5. Mulligan T, Frick MF, Zuraw QC, Stemhagen A, McWhirter C. Prevalence of hypogonadism in males aged at least 45 years:the HIM study. *IJCP* 2006:60(7); 762-769

6. Araujo AB, et al. Total Testosterone as a Predictor of Mortality in Men. The Endocrine Society 2005 Annual Meeting, San Diego, CA, June 4-7

7. Shores MM, Matsumoto AM, Sloan KL, et al., Low serum testosterone and mortality in male veterans, *Arch Intern Med* 2006;166:1660–65

8. Laughlin GA, Barrett-Connor E, Bergstrom J Low serum testosterone and mortality in older men. J Clin Endocrinol Metab 2008: 93 (1) 68-75

9. Wu FCW, Von Eckhardstein A. Androgens and coronary disease. *Endocr Rev* 2003; 24: 183-217

10. English KM, Mandour O, Steeds RP, Diver MJ, Jones TH, Channer KS. Men with coronary artery disease have lower levels of androgens than men with normal coronary angiograms. *Eur Heart J* 2000; 21: 890-4

11. Malkin CJ Pugh,PJ Jones TH, Channer KS. Testosterone for secondary prevention in men with ischaemic heart disease? *Q J Med* 2003; 96: 521-529

12. Dai WS, Gutai JP, Kuller LH, Falvo-Gerard L. Relation between plasma high-density lipoprotein cholesterol and sex hormone concentrations in men. *Am J Cardiol* 1984; 53:1259–63

13. Phillips GB, Jing TY, Laragh JH et al. Serum sex hormone levels and Renin-sodium profile in men with hypertension. *Am J Hypertens* 1995; 8:626–9

14. Phillips GB, Jing TY, Resnick, Barbagallo M, Laragh JH, Sealey JE LM. Sex hormones and hemostatic risk factors for coronary heart disease in men with hypertension. *J Hypertens* 1993; 11:699–702

15. Haffner SM, Shaten J, Stern MP, Smith GD, Kuller L. Low levels of sex hormone-binding globulin and testosterone predict the development of non-insulin-dependent diabetes mellitus in men. MRFIT Research Group. Multiple Risk Factor Intervention Trial. *Am J Epidemiol.* 1996;143:889-897

16. English KM, Steeds RP, Jones TH, Diver MJ, Channer KS. Low-dose transdermal testosterone therapy improves angina threshold in men with chronic stable angina: a randomized, double-blind, placebo-controlled study. *Circulation* 2000; 102: 1906-11

17. Webb CM, McNeill JG, Hayward CS, de Zeigler D, Collins P. Effects of Testosterone on Coronary Vasomotor Regulation in men with Coronary Heart Disease. *Circulation* 1999; 100:1690–6

18. Hak AE, Witteman JCM, De Jong FH, et al., Low levels of endogenous androgens increase the risk of atherosclerosis in elderly men: the Rotterdam Study, *J Clin Endocrinol Metab*,2002;87:3632–9

19. Thompson IM, Tangen CM, Goodman PJ et al. Erectile dysfunction and subsequent cardiovascular disease. *JAMA* 2005: 294 (23): 2996-3002

20. Ma RCW, So WY, Yang XL et al. Erectile dysfunction predicts coronary heart disease in type 2 diabetes *J Am Coll Cardiol* 2008: 51 (21) 2045- 2050

21. Gazzaruso C, Solerte SB, Pujia A et al. Erectile dysfunction as a predictor of cardiovascular events and death in diabetic patients with angiographically proven asymptomatic coronary artery disease. *J Am Coll Cardiol* 2008: 51 (21) 2040- 2044

22. Khaw KT, Dowsett M, Folkerd E et al.Endogenous testosterone and mortality due to all causes, cardiovascular disease, and cancer in men: European Prospective Investigation into Cancer in Norfolk (EPIC-Norfolk) prospective population study. *Circulation* 2007: 116 (23) 2694- 2701

23. OhJY, Barrett-Connor E, Wedick NM, Wingard DL; Rancho Bernardo Study. Endogenous sex hormones and the development of type 2 diabetes in older men and women; the Rancho Bernardo study. *Diabetes Care.* 2002; 25: 55-60

24. Phillips GB, Pinkernell BH, Jing TY. The association of hypotestosteronemia with coronary artery disease in men. *Arterioscler Thromb* 1994:14 (5): 701-6

25. Rosano GMC, Sheiban I, Massaro R et al. Low testosterone levels are associated with coronary artery disease in male patients with angina. *Int J Impot Res* 2007:19 (2) 176- 182

26. Pugh PJ, Morris PD, Hall J et al. High prevalence of low testosterone levels in men with coronary heart disease and an association with hypertension and obesity - The South Yorkshire study. *Endocrine Abstracts* 2003: 5: 225

27. Murphy S, Kham ST, Cassidy A. Compston JE. Sex Hormones and bone mineral density in elderly men. *Bone miner* 1993; 20: 133-140

28. NICE guidance on Osteoporosis www.nice.org.uk

29. NICE guidance on prostate cancer. www.nice.org.uk

30. Rudman D, Drinka PJ, Wilson CR, Mattson DE, Scherman F, Cuisinier MC, Relations of endogenous anabolic hormones and physical activity to bone mineral density and lean body mass in elderly men. *Clin Endocrinol* 1994; 40: 653-661

31. Buvat J, Boujadoue G. Testosterone replacement in the ageing male. *J Men's Health and Gender.* 2005;2:396-399

32. Wang BC, Cunningham G, Dobs A, Iranmanesh A et al. Long term testosterone gel treatment maintains beneficial effects on sexual function, lean and fat mass, and bone mineral density in hypogonadal men. *J Clin Endocrinol Metab* 2004; 89: 2085-2098

33. Fonda S, Bertrand R, O'Donnell A, Longcope C, Mc Kincley JB. Age, hormones and cognitive function among middle-aged and elderley men: cross sectional evidence from the Massachusetts Male Ageing study. *J Gerontology* 2005; 60A: 385-390

34. Barrett-Connor E, Goodman-Gruen G, Patay B. Endogenous sex hormones and cognitive function in older men. *J Clin Endocrin Metab* 1999; 84: 3861-3685

35. Moffat SD, Zonderman AB, Metter EJ, Blackman MR, Harman SM. Resnick SM. Longitudinal assessment of serum free testosterone concentration predicts memory performance and cognitive status in elderly men. *J Clin Endocrinol Metab* 2002; 87: 5001-5007

36. Kaufman JM, Vermeulen A. The decline in androgen levels in androgen levels and its clinical and therapeutic implications. *Endocrine Rev* 2005; 26; 833-876

37. Goldney R, Phillips P, et al. (2004). Diabetes, depression and quality of life: A population study. *Diabetes Care,* 27(5): 1066-70

38. Anderson RJ, Freedland KE, et al. (2001). The prevalence of co-morbid depression in adults with diabetes: a meta-analysis.*Diabetes Care,* 24(6): 1069-78

38. Lustman PJ, Anderson RJ, et al. (2000). Depression and poor glycaemic control: a meta-analytic review of the literature. *Diabetes Care,* 23(7): 934-42

39. Quality and Outcome framework guidance for GMS contract 2008/09 – NHS Employers. www.nhsemployers.org

40. Kapoor D, Goodwin E, Channer KS, Jones TH, et al.,Testosterone replacement therapy improves insulin resistance, glycaemic control, visceral adiposity and hypercholesterolemia in hypogonadal men with Type 2 diabetes, *Eur J Endocrinol,* 2006;154:899–906

41. Naharci MI, Pinar M, Bolu E, Olgun A. Effect of testosterone on insulin sensitivity in men with idiopathic hypogonadotropic hypogonadism. *Endocr Pract.* 2007 ;13: 629-635

References

42. Boyanov MA, Boneva Z, Christov VG, Testosterone supplementation in men with type 2 diabetes, visceral obesity and partial androgen deficiency, *Aging Male*, 2003;6:1–7

43. Jones T.. A Placebo Controlled Study on the Effects of Transdermal Testosterone Gel in Hypogonadal Men With Type II Diabetes or Metabolic Syndrome in Diabetic Control and Insulin Sensitivity: The TIMES 2 Study. Abstract P3-422

44. Pope HG, Cohane GH, Kanayama G, Siegel AJ, Hudson JL. Testosterone gel supplementation for men with refractory depression. A randomised placebo controlled study. *Am J Psychiatry* 2003; 160: 105-111

45. Moffat SD et al, Free Testosterone and risk for Alzheimer disease in older men, *Neurology*, 2004, 62 (2): 188-93

46. Hogervorst E et al, Low free testosterone is an independent risk factor for Alzheimer's disease, *Exp Gerontol* 2004, 39 (11-12), 1633

47. Carani C, Isidori AM, Granata A, et al. Multicentre study of sexual symptoms in male hypo and hyperthyroid patients. *J Endo Crin Metab* 2005; 90: 6472-6479

48. Vermeulen A. Androgen replacement therapy in the ageing male - a critical evaluation. *J Clin Endocrinol Metab* 2001; 86: 2380-90

49. Buvat J, Boujadoue G. Testosterone replacement therapy in the ageing male. *J Men's Health and Gender* 2005; 2: 396-399

50. Roden EL, Morgentale et al. Risks of testosterone replacement therapy and recommendations for monitoring. *New Eng Journal of Medicine* 2004; 350: 482-492

51. Shabsigh R. Testosterone and ED. *J Sex Med* 2005; 2: 6 785-792

52. Kalinchenko SY, Kozlov GI, Gontcharov NP, Katsiya GV. Oral testosterone undecanoate reverses erectile dysfunction associated with diabetes mellitus in patients failing on sildenafil citrate therapy alone. *Aging Male.* 2003; 6: 94-99

53. Shabsigh R et al. Therapy with Testosterone gel 1% improves response to Sildenafil in erectile dysfunction. *J Urol* 2004; 172: 658-663

54. Kapoor D, Aldred H, Clark S, et al., Clinical and biochemical assessment of hypogonadism in men with type 2 diabetes, Correlations with bioavailable testosterone and visceral adiposity, *Diabetes Care,* 2007;30:911–17

55. Laaksonen De et al. Testosterone and sex hormone binding globulin predict the metabolic syndrome in middle aged men. Diabetes Care 2004; 27: 103656. 13. Andersson B, Marin P, Lissner L, et al., Testosterone concentrations in women and men with NIDDM, *Diabetes Care,* 1994;17:405–11

57. Dhindsa S, Prabhakar S, Sethi M. et al., Frequent occurrence of hypogonadotrophic hypogonadism in type 2 diabetes, *J Clin End Metab,* 2004;89:5462–8

58. Isidori AM, Strollo F,Morè M, Caprio M, Aversa A, Moretti A, Leptin and Aging: Correlation with Endocrine Changes in Male and Female Healthy Adult Populations of Different Body Weights *The Journal of Clinical Endocrinology & Metabolism* Vol. 85, No. 5 1954-1962

59. P Cohen The hypogonadal–obesity cycle: role of aromatase in modulating the testosterone–estradiol shunt – a major factor in the genesis of morbid obesity. *Medical Hypotheses*, 1999 Volume 52, Issue 1 , Pages 49 - 51

60. Hackett G, Cole N, Deshpande A, Popple M, Kennedy D. Biochemical associations of testosterone and type 2 diabetes. Poster ESSM Brussels Dec 2008

61. Quality and Outcomes Framework Guidance for GMS contract 2008/9 June 2008. www.nhsemployers.com

62. NICE guidance on type 2 diabetes. www.nice.org.uk

63. Stratton IM, Adler AI, Neil HA, et al. Association of glycaemia with macrovascular and microvascular complications of type 2 diabetes (UKPDS 35): prospective observational study. *BMJ* 2000;321:405-412

64. Holman R et al. 10 year follow-up of Intensive Glucose Control in Type 2 Diabetes. *N Engl J Med* 2008 Published on-line Sept 10th 2008

65. Patel A, MacMahon S, Chalmers J, et al. Effects of a fixed combination of perindopril and indapamide on macrovascular and microvascular outcomes in patients with type 2 diabetes mellitus (the ADVANCE trial): a randomised controlled trial. *Lancet* 2007;370:829-840

66. The Action to Control Cardiovascular Risk in Diabetes Study Group. Effects of intensive glucose lowering in type 2 diabetes. *N Engl J Med* 2008;358:2545-2559

67. Nieshlag E, Behre H, Bouchard P, et al., Testosterone replacement therapy: current trends and future directions, *Hum Reprod Update*, 2004;5:409–1.

68. Rhoden EL, Ribeiro EP, Riedner CE, Teloken C, Souto CA. Glycosylated haemoglobin levels and the severity of erectile function in diabetic men. *BJU Int.* 2005;95:615-617

69. Romeo JH, Seftel AD, Madhun ZT, Aron DC. Sexual function in men with diabetes type 2: association with glycemic control. *J Urol.* 2000;163:788-791

70. Jones T. A Placebo Controlled Study on the Effects of Transdermal Testosterone Gel in Hypogonadal Men with Type II Diabetes or Metabolic Syndrome in Diabetic Control and Insulin Sensitivity: The TIMES 2 Study. Abstract P3-422

71. Heufelder A. Testosterone gel improves parameters in type 2 diabetes. Satellite symposium. ESSM Vienna, 2006

72. The Endocrine Society. Clinical bulletins in andropause: benefits and risks of treating hypogonadism in the ageing male. *Endocr Rep* 2002; 2: 1-6

73. Roden E Morgentaler A. Rules of Testosterone replacement and recommendations for monitoring. *NEJM* 2004; 350: 384-392

74. Porst H, Buvat J, Standard Practice in Sexual Medicine. 2006. www.blackwellpublishing.co.uk

75. Schubert M, Minnemann T et al. Intramuscular testosterone undecanoate: pharmacokinetic aspects of a novel testosterone formulation during long term treatment for men with hypogonadism. *J Clin Endocrin Metab* 2004; 89: 5429-5434

76. Goren L, Mathijas C. Transdermal testosterone delivery. *World J Urol* 2003;21:316-319

77. McNicholas TA, Dean JD, Mulder H, Carnegie C, Jones NA. A novel testosterone gel formulation normalizes androgen levels in hypogonadal men, with improvements in body composition and sexual function. *BJU Int* 2003; 91: 69-74

78. Bhasin S, Singh AB, Mac RP, Carter B, Lee MI, Cunningham GR. Managing the risks of prostate disease during testosterone replacement therapy in older men: recommendations for a standardized monitoring plan. *Journal of Andrology* 2003; 24:3 299-311

79. Morales A. Androgen replacement therapy and prostate safety. *Eur Urol* 2002; 41:113-20

80. The Endocrine Society. Clinical bulletins in andropause: benefits and risks of treating hypogonadism in the ageing male. *Endocr Rep* 2002; 2: 1-6

81. Philip J, Dutta Roy S, Ballal M, Foster CS, Javle P. Is a digital rectal examination necessary in the diagnosis and clinical staging of early prostate cancer? *BJU Int* 2005; 95:969-71

82. Morgentaler A, Bruning CO 3rd, DeWolf WC. Occult prostate cancer in men with low serum testosterone levels. *JAMA* 1996; 276:1904-6

83. Schatzl G ,Madersbacher S Thurridl T, Waldmüller J, Kramer J, Haitel A, Marberger M, High-grade prostate cancer is associated with low serum testosterone levels. *Prostate* 2001 Vol47 Issue 1, Pages 1 - 75 (1 April 2001)

84. Schatzl G, Madersbacher S, Haitel A, Gsur A, Preyer M, Haidinger G, et al. Associations of serum testosterone with microvessel density, androgen receptor density and androgen receptor gene polymorphism in prostate cancer. *J Urol* 2003; 169:1312-1317

85. Massengill JC, Sun L, Moul JW, Wu H, McLeod DG, Amling C, et al. Pretreatment total testosterone level predicts pathological stage in patients with localized prostate cancer treated with radical prostatectomy. *J Urol* 2003; 169:1670-5

86. Imamoto T, Suzuki H, Fukasawa S, Shimbo M, Inahara M, Komiya A, et al. Pretreatment serum testosterone level as a predictive factor of pathological stage in localized prostate cancer patients treated with radical prostatectomy. *Eur Urol* 2005; 47:308-12

87. Hajjar RR, Kaiser FF, Morley JE. Outcomes of long term testosterone replacement in older hypogonadal males: a retrospective analysis. *J endocrinol metabolism* 1997;82:3793-3796

88. Morales A. Androgen replacement therapy and prostate safety. *Eur Urol* 2002;41:113-1120

89. R Shabsigh, E D Crawford, A Nehra, and K M Slawin Testosterone therapy in hypogonadal men and potential prostate cancer risk: a systematic review International Journal of Impotence Research advance online publication 17 July 2008; doi: 10.1038/ijir.2008.31

90. Agarwal PK, Oefelein MG. Testosterone replacement therapy after primary treatment for prostate cancer. *J Urol* 2005; 173:533-6

91. Porst H, Broemel T, Hyperprolactinaemia in men with sexual dysfunction. Still a diagnostic challenge. *J Sex Med* 2006;3 (suppl 1);53

92. Buvat J, Boujaoude G. Hyperprolactinaemia et function sexuelle chez l'homme. *Androlgie* 2005 ;15 :366-373

93. Molitch ME. Medication induced hyperprolactinaemia. *Mayo Clin Proc* 2005;82:1050-1057

94. De Rosa M, Zarrilli S, Di Sarno A, Hyperprolactinaemia in men. *Endocrine* 2003;20:75-82

95. American Psychiatric association. Diagnostic and Statistical Manual of Mental Disorders, 3rd edition. Washington DC. 1980

96. Kaplan HS. The sexual desire disorders: dysfunctional regulation of sexual motivation. New York: Brunner/Mazel, 1995

97. Levine SB. The Nature of Sexual Desire. A clinician's Perspective. *Arch Sex Behav* 2003; Jun 32 (3): 279-285

98. Meuleman EJ,Van Lankvled J. Hypoactive Sexual Desire Disorder: an underestimated condition in men. *BJU Int* 2005; 95: 201-296

99. Laumann EO, Paik A, Rosen RC, Sexual Dysfunction in the United States. Prevalence and predictors. *JAMA* 1999; 281 (6): 537-544

100. Wadsworth J, J Field, AM Johnson, S Bradshaw, K Wellings, Methodology of the National Survey of Sexual Attitudes and Lifestyles. *J R Stat Soc Ser A Stat Soc* 1993;156:407-421

101. Laumann EO, Nicolosi A, Glasser DB, Paik A, Ginge C. Sexual problems among men and women aged 40-80yrs. Prevalence and correlates identified in the Global Study of sexual attitudes and behaviours. *Int J Imp Res* 2005; 17: 39-57

102. Meston CM, Frohlich PE. The neurology of sexual function. *Arch Gen Psychiatry* 2000: 57: 1012-1030

103. Cutler WB, Friedmann E, McCoy NL. Pheromonal influences on sociosexual behaviour in men. *Arch Sex Behav* 1998; 27: 1-13

104. Montejo-Gonzalez AL, LLorca G, Izquierdo JA et al. SSRI induced dysfunction: fluoxetine, paroxetine, sertraline and fluvoxamine in a prospective multicentre and descriptive clinical study of 344 patients. *J Sex Marital Ther* 1997; 23: 176-193

105. White JM, Rumbold GR, Behavioral effects of Histamine and its antagonists:a review Psychopharmacology 1988: 85: 1-1462. Hoyl MT, Alessi CA, Harker JO, Development and testing of the five-item geriatric depression scale in elderly subjects in three different settings. *J Am Geriatric Soc* 1999; 47: 873-878

106. Coruna G, Mannucci E, Petrone L, Glommi R, Mansani R et al. Psycho-biological correlates of hypoactive sexual desire in patients with erectile dysfunction. *Int J Imp Res* 2004; 16: 275-281

107. Gelenberg AJ, MacGahuey C, Laukes C, et al. Mirtazapine substitution in SSRI-induced sexual dysfunction. *J Clin Psychiatry* 2000; May 61 (5): 356-360

108. Ferris RM, Cooper BR, Maxwell RA. Studies of Bupropion's mechanism of antidepressant activity. *J Clin Psychiact* 1983; 44: 74-78

109. Pyke R, Goldfischer et al, The safety and tolerability of Flibanserin in premenopausal women with hypoactive sexual desire disorder (HSDD) Poster NR5-115. American College of OBGYN 2008

110. Leiblum S, Rosen R. Principles and Practice of Sex Therapy 3rd Edition Guildford Press New York

111. Shifren JL, Davis SR, Moreau M, Waldbaum A, Bouchard C, DeRogatis L, Derzko C, Bearnson P, Kakos N, O'Neill S, Levine S, Wekselman K, Buch A, Rodenberg C, Kroll R. Testosterone patch for the treatment of hypoactive sexual desire disorder in naturally menopausal women: results from the INTIMATE NM1 Study: *Menopause.* 2006 Sep-Oct;13(5):770-9

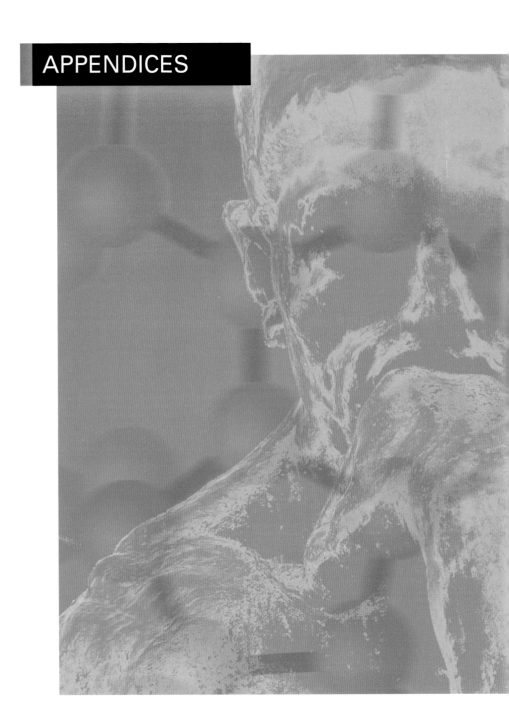

APPENDICES

The Role of Androgens in Men's Health

APPENDIX 1

Nomogram for calculating free testosterone from total testosterone and SHBG

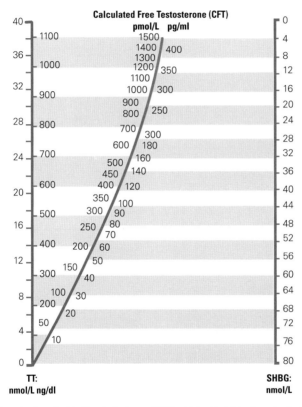

Calculated Free Testosterone (CFT)

The value for calculated free testosterone (CFT) is obtained by joining the value for TT to that for SHBG and where the line intersects the middle curved scale is the value for CFT. The figure is derived from the equation given by Vermeulen A. Verdonck L, Kaufman JM. A critical evaluation of simple methods for the estimation of free testosterone in serum. *J Clin Endocrinol Metab* 1999;84:3666-72. An average albumin value of 43 g/l is assumed, though unless there are markedly lower levels due to malnutrition or immobilization, changes in this variable make little difference.

© M. Carruthers, ADAM: Androgen Deficiency in the Adult Male, Taylor & Francis, 2004

Appendices

APPENDIX 2

Algorithm for treating Testosterone Deficiency Syndrome

based on the EAU, ISA and ISSAM* recommendations[1]

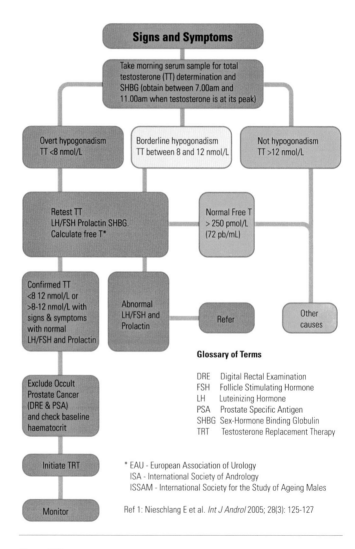

Signs and Symptoms

Take morning serum sample for total testosterone (TT) determination and SHBG (obtain between 7.00am and 11.00am when testosterone is at its peak)

| Overt hypogonadism TT <8 nmol/L | Borderline hypogonadism TT between 8 and 12 nmol/L | Not hypogonadism TT >12 nmol/L |

Retest TT LH/FSH Prolactin SHBG. Calculate free T*

Normal Free T > 250 pmol/L (72 pb/mL)

Confirmed TT <8 12 nmol/L or >8-12 nmol/L with signs & symptoms with normal LH/FSH and Prolactin

Abnormal LH/FSH and Prolactin

Refer

Other causes

Exclude Occult Prostate Cancer (DRE & PSA) and check baseline haematocrit

Initiate TRT

Monitor

Glossary of Terms

DRE   Digital Rectal Examination
FSH   Follicle Stimulating Hormone
LH   Luteinizing Hormone
PSA   Prostate Specific Antigen
SHBG   Sex-Hormone Binding Globulin
TRT   Testosterone Replacement Therapy

* EAU - European Association of Urology
 ISA - International Society of Andrology
 ISSAM - International Society for the Study of Ageing Males

Ref 1: Nieschlang E et al. *Int J Androl* 2005; 28(3): 125-127

APPENDIX 3

The International Index of Erectile Function

Over past 4 weeks:

Q1. How often were you able to get an erection during sexual activity?

0 = No sexual activity
1 = Almost never/never
2 = A few times (much less than half the time)
3 = Sometimes (about half the time)
4 = Most times (much more than half the time)
5 = Almost always/always

Q2. When you had erections with sexual stimulation, how often were your erections hard enough for penetration?

0 = No sexual activity
1 = Almost never/never
2 = A few times (much less than half the time)
3 = Sometimes (about half the time)
4 = Most times (much more than half the time)
5 = Almost always/always

Q3. When you attempted sexual intercourse, how often were you able to penetrate (enter) your partner?

0 = Did not attempt intercourse
1 = Almost never/never
2 = A few times (much less than half the time)
3 = Sometimes (about half the time)
4 = Most times (much more than half the time)
5 = Almost always/always

Appendices

Q4. During sexual intercourse, how easily were you able to maintain your erection after you had penetrated (entered) your partner?

0 = Did not attempt intercourse
1 = Extremely difficult
2 = Very difficult
3 = Difficult
4 = Slightly difficult
5 = Not difficult

Q5. During sexual intercourse, how difficult was it to maintain your erection to completion of intercourse?

0 = Did not attempt intercourse
1 = Extremely difficult
2 = Very difficult
3 = Difficult
4 = Slightly difficult
5 = Not difficult

Q6. How many times have you attempted sexual intercourse?

0 = No attempts
1 = One to two attempts
2 = Three to four attempts
3 = Five to six attempts
4 = Seven to 10 attempts
5 = More than 11 attempts

Q7. When you attempted sexual intercourse, how often was it satisfactory to you?

0 = Did not attempt intercourse
1 = Almost never/never
2 = A few times (much less than half the time)
3 = Sometimes (about half the time)
4 = Most times (much more than half the time)
5 = Almost always/always

Q8. How much have you enjoyed sexual intercourse?

0 = No intercourse
1 = No enjoyment
2 = Not very enjoyable
3 = Fairly enjoyable
4 = Highly enjoyable
5 = Very highly enjoyable

Q9. When you had sexual stimulation or intercourse, how often did you ejaculate?

0 = No sexual stimulation/intercourse
1 = Almost never/never
2 = A few times (much less than half the time)
3 = Sometimes (about half the time)
4 = Most times (much more than half the time)
5 = Almost always/always

Q10. When you had sexual stimulation or intercourse, how often did you have the feeling of orgasm or climax?

0 = No sexual stimulation/intercourse
1 = Almost never/never
2 = A few times (much less than half the time)
3 = Sometimes (about half the time)
4 = Most times (much more than half the time)
5 = Almost always/always

Q11. How often have you felt sexual desire?

1 = Almost never
2 = A few times (much less than half the time)
3 = Sometimes (about half the time)
4 = Most times (much more than half the time)
5 = Almost always/always

Q12. How would you rate your level of sexual desire?

1 = Very low/none at all
2 = Low
3 = Moderate
4 = High
5 = Very high

Q13. How satisfied have you been with your overall sex life?

1 = Very dissatisfied
2 = Moderately dissatisfied
3 = About equally satisfied and dissatisfied
4 = Moderately satisfied
5 = Very satisfied

Q14. How satisfied have you been with your sexual relationship with your partner?

1 = Very dissatisfied
2 = Moderately dissatisfied
3 = About equally satisfied and dissatisfied
4 = Moderately satisfied
5 = Very satisfied

Q15. How do you rate your confidence that you could get and keep an erection?

1 = Very low
2 = Low
3 = Moderate
4 = High
5 = Very high

Six questions (1-5, 15) are related to erectile function,
three (6-8) to satisfaction with intercourse,
two (9, 10) to orgasm,
two (11, 12) to sexual desire,
and two (13, 14) to overall satisfaction
A score of 25 or less is consistent with erectile dysfunction.

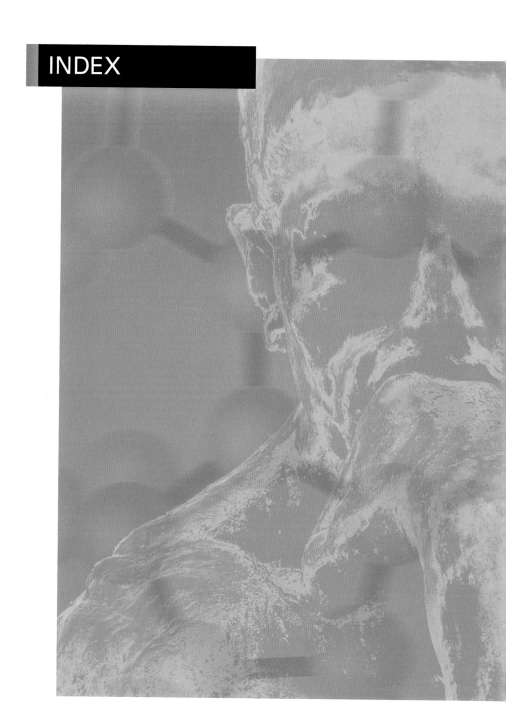

INDEX

A

ACCORD study 39
ADVANCE Study 39
Alzheimer's disease 24
Anaemia 20, 24
Androgen deficiency of the
    ageing male (ADAM) 5, 109
Androgen receptor
    polymorphism 22
Antipsychotics 66

B

Bone Mineral Density
    (BMD) 18
Bromocriptine 66, 85
BSSM 5, 57, 67

C

Cabergolide 66
Cardiovascular
    disease 9, 12, 13, 14, 39,
    41, 65, 68, 94
Chlorpromazine 66
Cognitive function 5, 20,
    24, 48, 52

D

Depression 22, 23, 48, 52, 74,
    77, 79, 80, 86, 87, 91, 93, 96
Dyslipidaemia 6, 94

E

EPIC study 11, 13
Erectile dysfunction
    (ED) 27, 36, 42, 58, 74,
    76, 80, 83, 86
Erythrocytosis 24
European Urology
    Association 57

F, G

Global Sexual Attitudes and
    Behaviours Study (GSSAB) 74

H

HDL cholesterol 9, 12
HIM study 6, 32, 51
Hypothyroidism 25, 67, 76, 78
Hyperthyroidism 25, 67, 76
Hyperprolactinaemia 25, 49,
    50, 65-66, 85
Hypogonadism 4, 5, 6, 8, 15,
    17, 20, 22, 25-27, 31-33, 47-50,
    62, 65, 69, 79, 94, 96, 110

I, J, K

Insulin resistance 14, 22, 31,
    33, 35, 41-43
International Society for
    the Ageing Male 77, 110